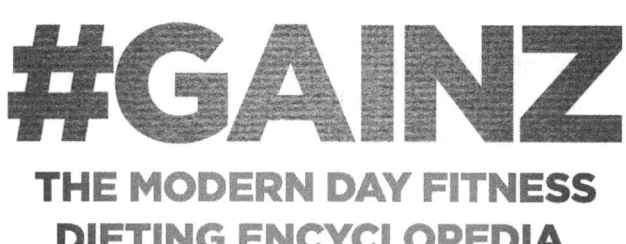

THE MODERN DAY FITNESS
DIETING ENCYCLOPEDIA

JORDAN MILLER

DISCLAIMER

Please review the following User Agreement carefully before using the exercises in this book.

I strongly recommend that you consult with your physician before beginning any exercise program.

You should be in good physical condition to be able to participate in any of the exercises mentioned in this book.

I am not a licensed medical care provider and represent that I have no expertise in diagnosing, examining, or treating medical conditions of any kind, or in determining the effect of any specific exercise on a medical condition.

You should understand that when participating in any exercise or exercise program, there is the possibility of physical injury. If you engage in any exercise in this book, you agree that you do so at your own risk, are voluntarily participating in these activities, assume all risk of injury to yourself, and agree to release and discharge me, the writer, from any and all claims or causes of action, known or unknown, arising.

DEDICATION

When it comes to whom this book should be dedicated to, a lot of names pop up. First of all, I want to thank Mum for being Mum. She always believed I would eventually succeed no matter how many times I failed. I would like to thank Dad for helping me with a place to live when I had fallen on my face.

I thank all of my followers that have supported me through the bright and the dark. I would like to dedicate this book to everyone who ever thought that dieting was hard. I would like to dedicate this book to everyone who got lost in the vast universe of the health and nutrition industry.

I dedicate this book to all people who are looking to finally take that leap; become educated, become motivated, and become a stronger, leaner, sharper, more powerful version of themselves.

To the 16-year-old kid who's a hard gainer and needs to learn how to properly bulk, this book is for you. To the 30-year-old mom who needs a practical blueprint to dieting for her physical and personal goals, this book is for you. For the 45-year-old obese person with little hope of ever looking and feeling different, this book is for you. For the 21-year-old who is looking to get into bodybuilding or any sort of physique show, this book is for you.

To that person reading this who doubts themselves, I don't doubt you, you can win. This book will get you into the mind frame to win at fitness and life.

I created this book to be the most relevant and current doctrine of modern dieting structure, protocol, and strategy.

From both a psychological and physical standpoint, this book is dedicated to helping you not only understand how food works on a deeper level than any other book on the market, but also to helping you get mentally prepared to take massive action.

Yes, there are many other highly technical diet and nutrition books on the market. There are many other fitness motivation books on the market as well, even 'how to' fitness books. But never has there been a book with all three elements, dedicated to introducing you to a complete guide to dieting in its entirety.

This book is dedicated to the person who is ready to change, and looking to put in the work to get there.

To be completely honest, it doesn't matter what you look like now. What matters most is where you're going, and finding the most efficient and effective means of getting there. This book is dedicated to helping you do that in the most effective and direct way possible.

ANYONE CAN DO THIS

I'm Jordan. I am here to tell you that eating to get shredded and build muscle is very simple. This book is dedicated to anyone who thinks that dieting is difficult. Whether you are a 16-year-old hard gainer looking to pack on the size, a 35-year-old looking to shred down, or a 65-year-old looking to build lean muscle and lose some fat, it isn't complicated.

You see, from the outside there is so much information and data on dieting, and it's thrown all over the place like paint splatter on a white wall. The truth is simplicity; the ultimate form of sophistication.

You may have a lot to learn, but once you develop a structure, strategy and method, it all happens very fast and ooh so easy.

I have been training and living the health and fitness lifestyle for almost eleven years, and I have tried almost every diet program you could imagine, including all of the popular fad diets. I've also tried all of the bizarre food and food timing manipulation techniques.

I'm not a scientist, but I do know what works and what will waste your time.

MY BREAKING POINT

It all started for me at 12 years old. I was a fat, out of shape, middle school kid who was picked on by everyone and called "faggot."

Bear in mind, I am straight. That is merely a word that close minded people used to describe those who were different in middle school.

I began getting picked on more and more, getting in fights every couple of days. This needed to end. I couldn't take it anymore. I was beginning to believe there was no hope for me and that all of the kids were right with their words.

This is when I would literally start getting sick at the thought of going back to school the next day. At this point, I was contemplating suicide. I had been working out a little, a couple days a week, but wasn't even sure if it was for me. At 13 years old, I was jumped and pretend raped in front of everyone. When the two bigger kids jumped on me, I went down awkwardly, my right leg twisted back and shot up. It tore my right knee apart. The scene was pretty gross; nobody cared, and nobody helped me up.

This happened in the school gym. I hobbled all the way

to the other side of the school, laid down in the middle of the field and called my mom.

"Mom, just got jumped, my right leg is broken, can you come pick me up?"

I didn't cry, so somehow the police, the principal and school officials regarded me as "putting on." It was horse play, the officers said. They had no fucking idea of the mental agony I was in.

No, I didn't cry. Physical pain didn't even register in my head. All I could think of was how I wanted to die, and how I also wanted those two kids dead. For the next couple of months, I was bed ridden, playing Halo 3, drinking game fuel, and eating hot Cheetos and skittles.

I didn't really move very much for those three months. Because of this I dealt with muscle atrophy at a massive scale. At the same time, I was eating well over 3000 calories a day of complete junk food. I was dying from the inside out.

My uncle, whom I looked up to, passed away right around the same time. I remember thinking that it's an odd feeling being alive but feeling like you're already dead.

At age 13 and a half, I attempted suicide several times, but never went 100% through with it.

Two of the scariest things I ever did, that I can hardly believe I did now, were to play Russian Roulette with a revolver, and call 911 so the police would come to my house, while I was holding a loaded rifle; "suicide by police officer."

Those were dark times for me. But, I am still here.

There was one little 1% glimpse of hope that I held onto with everything I had.

Obviously, I was not meant to die. After several close encounters with death, I realized I could turn this around.

This was my moment. Sitting in my room, looking up at the ceiling, I realized, *I'm more than how I look and feel right now.*

There is something about me, something I need to do for the world, and somehow I am going to effect it in a positive way. I can't die yet, not at my own hands.

Fuck this, fuck all of the people that have made me feel this way, they will not win, I am not dead.

At that moment, I decided to become who I am today, I just didn't know it yet.

Here is what I looked like around the time I was jumped:

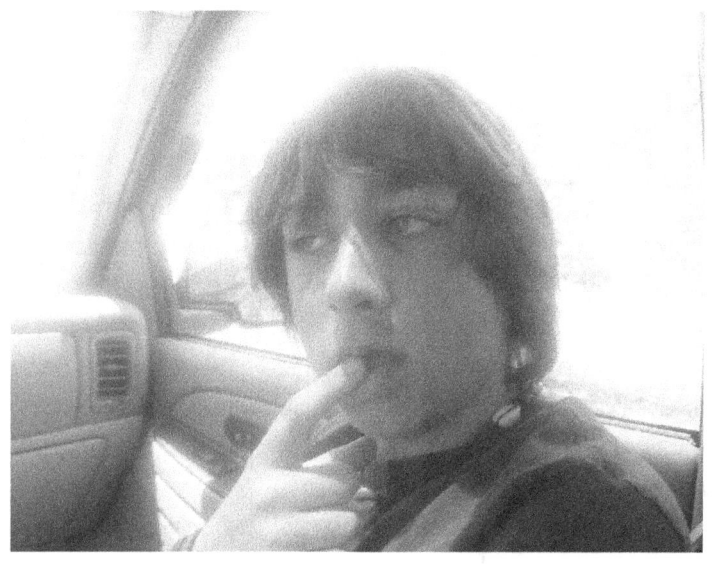

Attractive, right? I was one of those socially awkward, brainy kids. Here's another, just so you get the point.

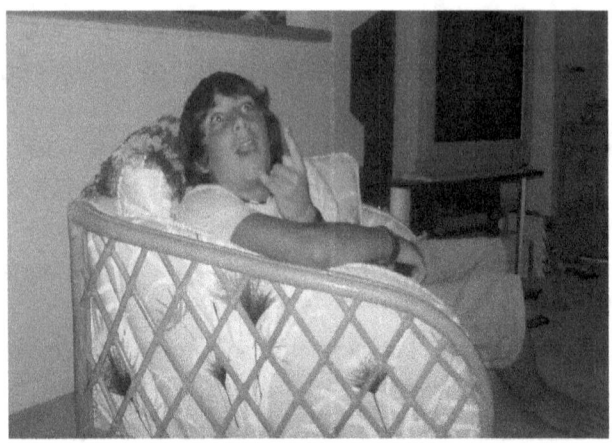

I believe you get the gist now. After I decided to become something, I carried myself with a fire in my eyes. I had nothing else to live for other than going to the gym and changing what I hated about myself. I began eating with more structure, paying attention to protein, and hitting the gym five days a week.

I was determined, and that determination came out of a very dark place. Because of this I am very resilient, the dark motivated me. This is what I looked like after a few years of intuitive eating and being consistent in the gym.

Not many people even realized I was the same kid from middle school that everybody picked on. I was never physically bullied again. I had developed a confidence - no-one fucked with me anymore.

These two years I not only trained bodybuilding-style, but I also worked on my cardiovascular, and mixed in some mixed martial arts training twice a week. I was 13 years old in the first two pictures and age fifteen in the last.

This picture of me was taken right after my first bodybuilding competition, where I placed 2nd in the teen division at only 15. The first place winner was 19 but turned 20 in just weeks after the comp, so he was basically 20.

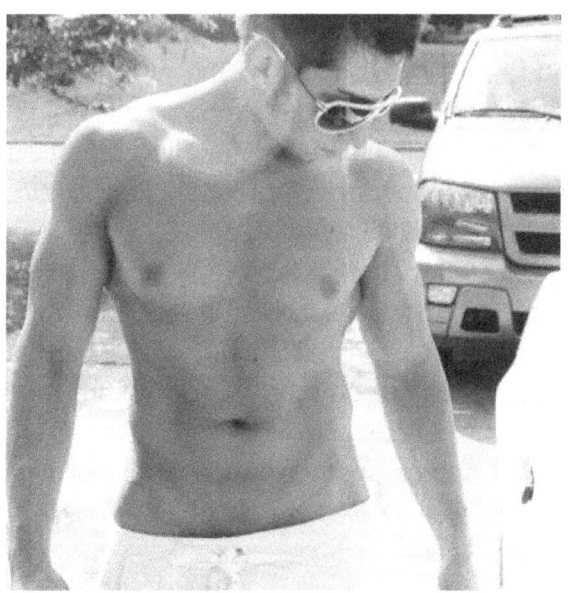

The Rebirth of Jordan

At age 15, I had thrown myself all in, and didn't even notice. I had already gone from a chubby, socially awkward nerd, to a confident teen bodybuilder. People weren't making fun of me anymore, they were looking up to me.

I loved it. It felt like I was becoming somebody that had the leverage to affect others in a positive way, it was a good time to be alive. Sadly, I was always very hard on myself and wasn't able to fully enjoy how far I had come in such a short time. I wanted to be much bigger, much leaner, and much stronger.

Up until this time, I had dieted. I went on a low carb diet to get like this. I lost nearly 40 pounds to achieve this look at age 15, and I was around 10% body fat in this picture. My abs just weren't really developed enough yet, plus my skin was a little loose from losing so much fat so quickly.

Shortly after I had already made a huge transformation, I decided to take this thing to the next level. I started reading, researching and learning everything about dieting. Around this time, I was starting to get questions every single day about how to get abs, or how to get big arms, or how to build muscle in general.

Basically, I become everyone's go-to diet and training coach, mostly diet. Diet was always much more interesting to me. It was so intriguing how carbs, fat and protein affected the body. I needed to learn more; what worked for me, what would work for others.

By 17, I had competed in three bodybuilding shows and placed well. Here are a couple more pics for progression's sake.

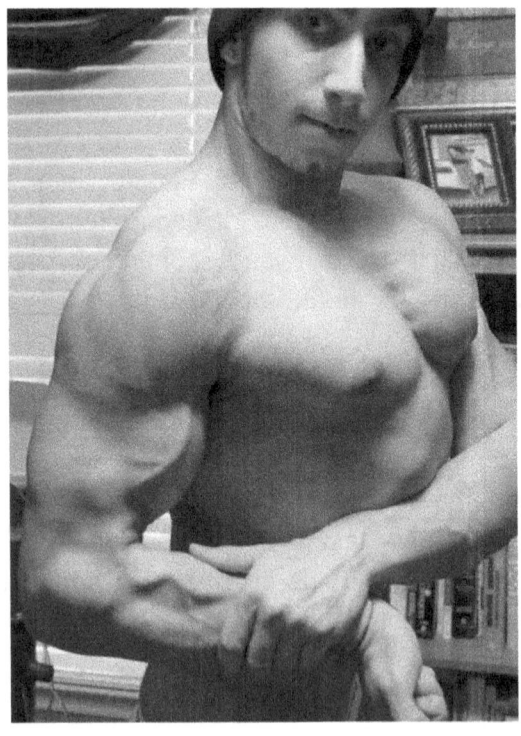

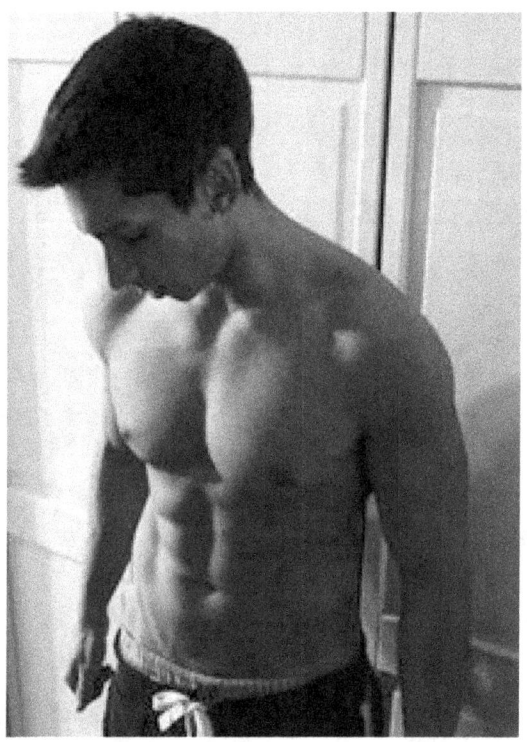

These two pictures of me were taken during contest prep for my second natural bodybuilding show. Between the ages of 16 and 18 I really began putting on some mass and learning how to maintain a lean physique while doing so. Here are two pictures of me at age 17.

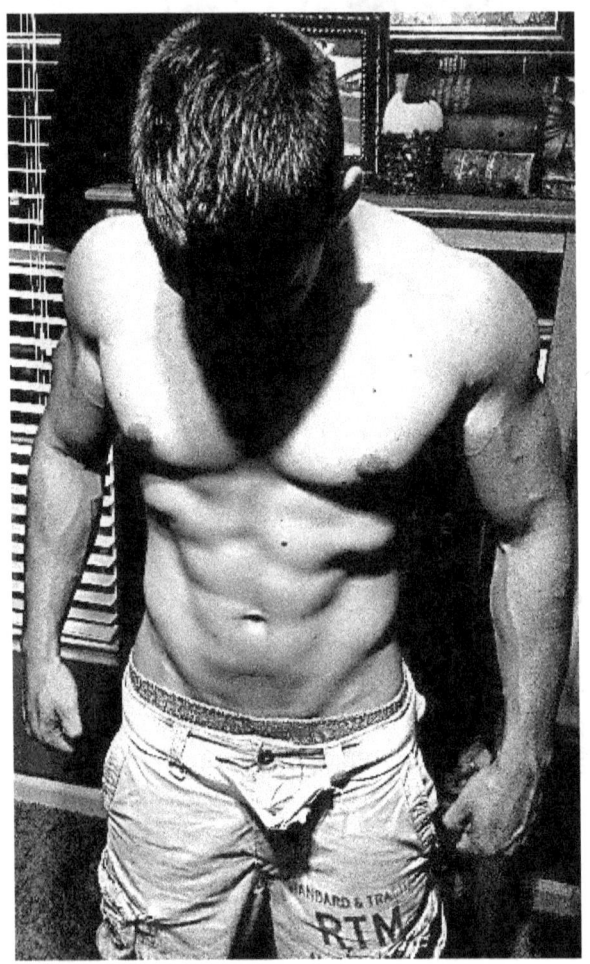

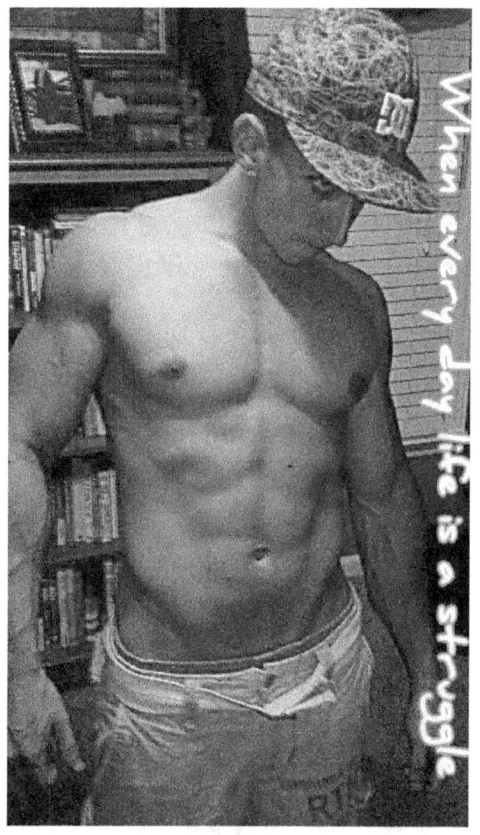

As you can see, I had built up my entire upper body pretty significantly. Deltoids, Traps, Chest, Arms, even my Abs had developed. This is around the time that I was first learning about IIFYM (If it fits your macros) and tracking macros. Before this, I simply dieted very bro for contest prep, and just ate intuitively when I wasn't prepping for a competition.

Learning about macros really opened my eyes and changed my life as a teen bodybuilder and coach. By 18 years old, I had already worked with an OCB Pro natural bodybuilder as my coach, as well as an IFBB Pro. By 18, I was really looking to start a career out of fitness, although I kind of already was doing it. This is the glimpse of light I saw at age 13; this is what was in my future that kept me from going through with suicide.

By 19, I had really transformed fitness into a career, and even took a liking to the film industry and acting. Imagine that: a kid who used to be socially awkward and anti-social is now a 19-year-old bodybuilder, actor, and entrepreneur. I doubt anyone could have predicted that, not even myself.

I began looking for my third bodybuilding coach at this time and hooked up with Jeff Alberts of Team 3DMJ. In case you aren't familiar, 3DMJ are regarded as some of the top natural bodybuilding coaches in the world. This was the icing on the cake. I got great at programming and macros, and was looking better than ever before. Here is a couple of pics of me at 19.

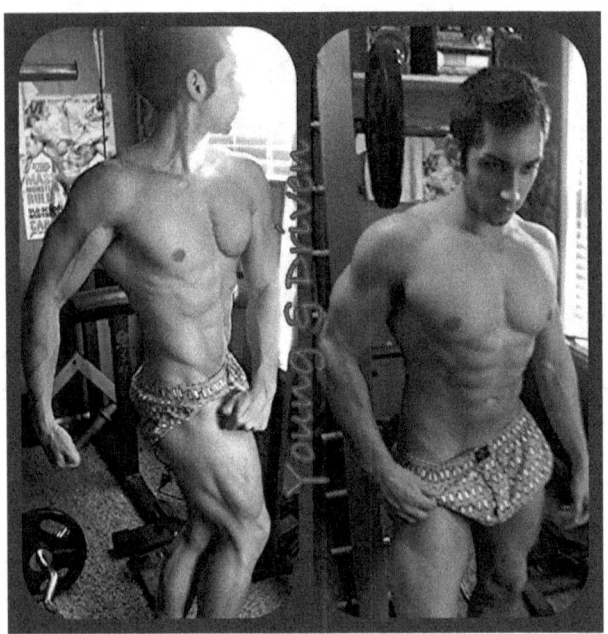

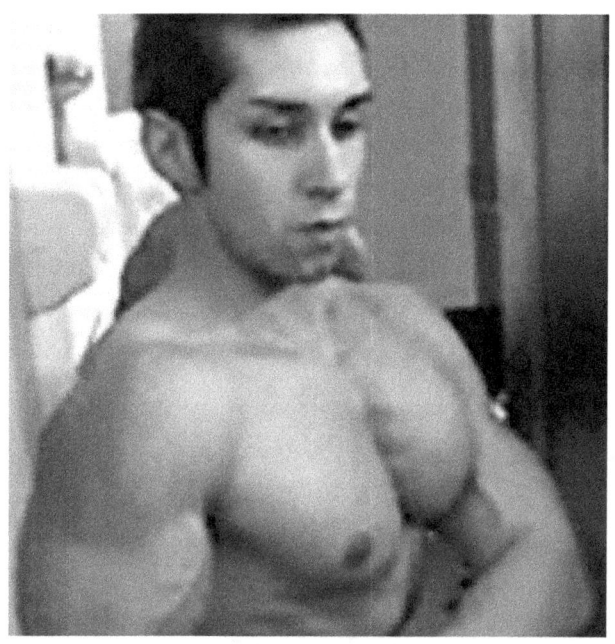

Around 18 or 19 years old, I had even decided to start a YouTube channel, and I still currently post 3-5 videos a week. This was what I was meant to do. This was why I was still alive.

This is really where I solidified fitness as a career. I had been coaching people and helping people since I was about 15, but now I was spending up to 8 hours a day working on YouTube and coaching.

I helped skinny guys pack on the mass by explaining to them the truth about food, their body and how they need to go about gaining mass. I helped overweight people go from overweight to shredded. I helped older people who had given up on themselves become more ripped and muscular then most 20-year-olds.

Hell, I even helped multiple girls get a booty. Getting a booty became such a thing I decided to write a small but powerful book series on Amazon coaching women on how to build the booty.

My goal had always been and will always be to help as many people as possible. This isn't my first fitness book, and I doubt it will be my last. I am 22 now. This is my life; I live to make your life better; I am here for you.

With over 10 years of dieting and training under my belt, 8 years of research, trial and error, and over 7 years of diet coaching, here I am today.

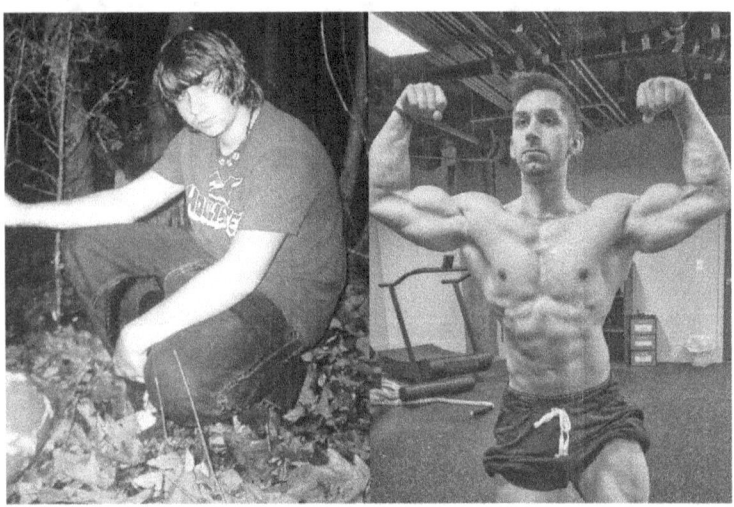

WHAT NOW?

I have really developed a passion for building a fitness brand using all of the skills that I've acquired over the years. Researching, writing, filming, acting, marketing, online coaching - that's what I'm up to these days.

I have 5 main goals with this book; 5 things that it must do for the world.

1. **Change the lives of 10 million people in the next 5 years.** That sounds epic, it's a challenge. If we can do it, and once it's done, I will make a fitness movie, the first of its kind. So mark my words, right now, if 10 million people purchase and change their lives from this book, there will be a movie. It will be on Netflix, you will be able to Netflix and chill while watching this movie.

2. **Change the way you see "diet."** Yes, 99% of the world thinks dieting is hard, militant, and makes life dull. They will never even try. Once those people finish this book, I want their minds to forever be opened. Living the fitness lifestyle complements your life, it doesn't make it more difficult.

3. **Light a Fire Under Your Ass.** Most people want to

look good, eat well, and be confident. The problem is, there is nothing pulling them towards these ideas. This book will light a fire under your ass so hot that it burns the laziness out of your soul. This is the moment you wake up, and you stop fucking saying *tomorrow* and run face forward into a better life. This is your moment to build that physique you have always wanted by learning how dieting actually works, and how seamless it can actually be.

4. **Start a Revolution.** Do you know how many diet fads and weight loss products are out there that waste our time and money? You buy them because of the way they were marketed to you, not for the results you won't receive. I am here to change your habits.

INTRODUCTION

There are a lot of diets out there. Thousands of methods from paleo dieting, to low fat, low carb, non-meat, non-diary, IIFYM, etc. It's really easy to get overwhelmed, and very easy to get lost with all of these contradicting methods and strategies.

Everyone has very biased diet philosophies all seemingly backed up by some study, which obviously makes their eating method the best, right? Nope, dieting from a practical standpoint is actually very simple, easily teachable, and not stressful and confusing. By reading this book you will understand "dieting" and the fact that dieting isn't really dieting.

If you really want to change your body and change your life, you need to learn the fundamentals of calories, fat, carbs, protein and micronutrients, and make them work for you. You need to learn what type of foods, the frequency, and what amounts work best for you taking into account your specific body type, your goals, and your relationship with food.

There is no 'one diet fits all'. Different people enjoy different forms of dieting, and different people need different ratios of fat, carbs and protein. The most important thing to consider is eating in a way that you enjoy, in a way that fits your lifestyle, and in a way that satisfies you and doesn't take time away from the things that matter in life, like work, your relationships and just in general things you don't need to obsess over.

You need to create a style of eating that coincides with your lifestyle and brings you toward your goals, not a diet that requires you to change your lifestyle to adapt to it.

Granted, some of you do actually need a full lifestyle overhaul. Whether you need a lifestyle overhaul or a way of eating that fits your lifestyle, you are about to learn exactly how to do both. I am taking it a step past just teaching you the how; I am also teaching you the what, the why, and the when.

Did you know that you can eat ice-cream, cookies, brownies and pancakes with blueberry breakfast syrup while getting shredded? Did you also know that there is a huge difference between something being healthy and calorically dense or low calorie?

I have spent over 10 years determining what works, for who, and why. I have also seen and experienced all of the things that don't work in the dieting & fitness world. I am going to share everything I know with you. By the time you finish this book, I promise you will not need any more information to start your healthy eating lifestyle, it's all here. If this book doesn't answer every single one of your dieting and lifestyle questions, return it.

CONTENTS

SECTION 1

MACRONUTRIENTS

Macronutrients are nutrients that provide your body with the energy it needs This energy is referred to as calories. These nutrients are necessary for growth, metabolism, and to maintain bodily functions. "Macro" means large, so macronutrients are nutrients needed in large amounts. There are three macronutrients: Carbohydrates (carbs), Fat, and Protein.

One gram of carbs contains **4** calories, one gram of fat contains **9** calories and one gram of protein contains **4** calories. I bolded these numbers so they would stand out in your head, you're welcome.

There is one other macronutrient, and most people don't realize that it even is a macronutrient, but it is. This macronutrient is not a carb, although people confuse it as being a carb a lot of the time. What I am talking about here is **alcohol.** Alcohol is its own separate macronutrient. So if you're wondering, yes technically there are 4 macronutrients.

The reason alcohol isn't normally regarded as one of the core macronutrients is that alcohol isn't part of your normal daily meals, for most of us. If alcohol is part of your daily meals, you my friend are an alcoholic and you need to deal with that before you worry about dieting or eating better.

Most food sources are a mix of fat/carb/protein. Since alcohol is made from the fermentation of grains, fruit, or vegetables, you won't find it in your normal unfermented foods, unless you batter your chicken in beer. You get my point: alcohol doesn't occur in a natural diet so it's not one of the 3 macros to hit every day.

CARBOHYDRATES

For most of you this is the most highly consumed macronutrient because Carbohydrates are needed in the largest amounts out of any of the 3 macronutrients. Your diet should be anywhere from between 40% to 65% carbs. Some people will fall close to 40% or even slightly lower, and some people will need many more carbs for energy.

These are the reasons we need carbohydrates.

- Carbohydrates are our bodies' main source of fuel.

- Carbs are easy for the body to break down and use as fuel.

- Carbs are made up of glucose and the body uses glucose to provide fuel for every cell and tissue in the body.

- Carbohydrates are needed for many bodily functions. You need carbs for your central nervous system, the kidneys, the brain, the muscles (even the heart) to function properly.

- Carbs can be stored in the muscles (you want

this), they can also be stored in the liver and later used as energy.

- Carbs are even important when it comes to intestinal health and waste elimination.

- The highest quantities of carbs are found in food sources such as starchy foods (like grains and potatoes), fruits, milk, and yogurt. Other foods like vegetables, beans, nuts, seeds and cottage cheese contain carbohydrates, but in much smaller amounts.

There is a certain type of carbohydrate that the body can't digest. Do you know what it is? Yep, its fiber. Fiber is a form of carbohydrate that the body cannot digest. These carbohydrates pass through the intestinal tract and help your body get rid of waste.

Not getting enough fiber can cause a slew of health problems like constipation and possibly colon cancer. Diets high in fiber help reduce the chance of heart disease, obesity, and they even help lower cholesterol.

Be careful though; too much fiber can irritate your gut and cause bad things to happen as well, like diarrhea. Nobody wants an uncontrollable anus in their life :(sad face). So now you're thinking, well I'm damned if I do, damned if I don't. Well, no, you're not.

The amount of fiber to shoot for is about 1 gram per 100 calories or 10 grams per 1000 calories. In some instances, 1.2 grams per 100 calories is ok; some people need more and some people need less. Generally sticking to around a gram of fiber per 100 calories is safe and healthy. You can get your fiber from fruits, vegetables, and whole grain products.

Demonizing carbs is stupid and unhealthy. Simply

put, some people function better with more or less carbs. Carbs aren't evil and carbs alone aren't responsible for fat gain, or prevention of fat loss. Carbs aren't the enemy, so don't listen to anyone that tells you to stop eating carbs, unless you personally feel better on a low carb diet, and some people do.

Even though your body uses carbs to do just about everything, it can use fat as well. Your body may be preset to function off of carbs, but fat can be used as fuel as well. It just takes some time for the body to adjust.

The point is, carbs are not evil, or your savior. They are simply one of the 3 macronutrients in food. For 90% of us, we function better using carbs as our main source of fuel, with protein for recovery and rebuilding the body, and fat as our bodies' secondary slow burning source of fuel.

The thing is, some people do feel better and perform better on fat based diets. My goal here is to help you become more open minded with food and dieting. There are ways to determine what works best for you and we will get into that later on in the book.

The 3 Different Levels of Carbs

So as intriguing as it sounds, carbs actually do break down into 3 different levels of molecules. People throw around the words "clean carbs" and "complex carbs" all the time to sound smart. The problem is that most of them don't understand what they're talking about.

See, a "dirty carb" is really just a simple sugar which is known as a Monosaccharide, which is basically a single carbohydrate. Simple carbs aren't "dirty carbs," they're just sugar carbs. The thing is, all carbs break down and metabolize just the same whether they are simple carbs or super complex carbs.

There are 3 different types of simple carbs: Glucose, Galactose, and Fructose. None of them are evil. Then we have a double molecule carbohydrate which is called a Disaccharide. There are 3 different types of disaccharides: Sucrose, Lactose, and Maltose. These forms of carbs are not evil either, just slightly more complex than a simple sugar. The third type of carb is known as the "Complex Carb" and it is a polysaccharide. These "complex carbs" are carbs with more than 2 molecules, so there is some complexity associated with these forms of carbs, hint: the word complex.

The 3 forms of complex carbs are: Starch, Fiber, and Glycogen. Yes, these are technically the "clean carbs" we are always speaking of, but the whole terminology of dirty and clean carbs is pure ignorance.

There are highly refined foods such as candy, but they aren't "dirty" they just have no nutritional value, so call them "empty" carbs. These carbs are just as empty as the feeling they give you 30 minutes after eating them, if you're overeating them. Candy is nothing more than a simple carb (Sucrose), to be exact.

So, let's forget about dirty carbs, clean carbs, good carbs, and bad carbs. Let's look at carbohydrates for what they really are, which is a form of energy; *our bodies' preferred source of energy*. I am going to break all of these carbs down and explain what each of them is, what they do, and why this knowledge will greatly benefit you.

Simple Carbs

These are the evil devil child of carbs in the media and on Dr. Oz. Rather than demonize and shame simple carbs, lets aim to understand them and find out where they fit into your life and diet. Let me show you how to look at them and how not to look at them.

The simple carb, or monosaccharide, is a form of carbohydrate that is known as the sugar molecule, which is the simplest form of carbohydrate. As I explained a moment ago, there are 3 forms of simple carbs: Glucose, Galactose, and Fructose. Let's look into each of them separately!

- **Glucose** is probably something you have only heard thrown around in the doctor's office, but its more than just a doctor's health measurement tool. It's an important and often misunderstood form of energy. Glucose is a natural sugar found in foods and it also goes by the name of dextrose, or even blood sugar.

  Glucose is a part of the calorie pool of most carb sources like fruit, honey and syrup. There's even glucose in grains, beans, veggies, and nuts. It's pretty easy to find this simple carb in weight gainer powders, sports drinks and also creatine-transport supplements.

  Creatine is an essential compound for energy production and muscle growth. We will talk more about creatine later, but for now, just know it is important for making gains and getting "jacked."

  All of these supplements and sports drinks are nothing more than glucose. Yes, now you know, most sports drinks and highly marketed creatine formula supplements are actually just "glucose +" products, sold at a high profit margin with a cool name. Basically, you're paying for convenience: the convenience of glucose + creatine, glucose + protein, and glucose isolated sports drinks infused with electrolytes.

Now there are some exceptions, but the point is that "supplements" most of the time are not worth their monetary value when you think about how much simple supplements and table sugar cost apart.

I digress, back to glucose, which by the way, is also present in soft drinks in the form of corn syrup. The problem with soft drinks is that just one has more simple sugar in it then the USDA recommends for your *whole day*. It's Ironic that soft drink companies are still doing so well.

We are blatantly told what is acceptable by the USDA's standards, and then marketed to with highly subliminal ads for soft drinks. I am not saying soft drinks are evil, I just want you to see what I see. Personally, I like a nice diet soda sometimes.

The body has 3 different ways of making use of glucose, let's take a look. Your body can burn glucose immediately within mitochondria, releasing carbon dioxide as well as water and energy. If your body doesn't need to burn the glucose immediately for fuel, it is converted by the liver or muscles into glycogen.

Muscle glycogen's sole purpose is to provide

energy only to muscles. Liver glycogen, on the other hand, can supply energy to any part of the body. When glucose is not burned in the mitochondria or shuttled into the liver or muscles, you ought to know what happens, you guessed it: "fat stores."

Glucose left over after glycogen saturation is converted to fat by the liver, and stored in adipose tissue around the body. The amount of fat build-up will depend on different variables, but the most constant variable will be total calories in vs. total calories out.

Does the person consistently consume more than they burn through activity? To be completely honest, throughout this book I am going to tell you this 100 different ways, with different applications. But here's a toast to the first time I say it. No seriously, take a toast, this is legit. I will wait until you take a toast. Weight loss or weight gain is all about thermodynamics. This means if you are on a caloric surplus (eating more than you burn with activity) you will be gaining weight.

So, every day that you are on a surplus you will be gaining weight; over time, this adds up. If you are on a caloric deficit (burning more fuel than the amount of food you take in), you will be losing weight. This means over time on a caloric deficit, things change, you get leaner.

Those are the basics of thermodynamics on a macro scale, "macro" meaning large. Glucose is actually what every single carb is going to be broken down into in order to enter the bloodstream.

So just know that every complex carb you eat will eventually become glucose in your bloodstream, then it will be burned, converted to glycogen or stored as body fat.

Your pancreas monitors these concentrations of glucose in your blood. In other words, your pancreas is your blood/glucose regulator. If blood glucose levels become too high, insulin is released. The insulin signals fat and muscle cells to absorb glucose.

This brings your blood glucose to normal levels and this is something that happens after every meal. On the contrary, if glucose levels are too low, "Glucagon" is released, which signals the liver to break down glycogen and release glucose to the blood. This raises your blood glucose level back to normal levels. This happens between meals.

- **Galactose** is another simple sugar and that's similar to glucose but has a different arrangement of atoms. The main source of galactose is lactose from milk and yogurt, which is one-part galactose and one-part glucose.

  Galactose is mostly absorbed into the liver, where it is mainly converted into liver glucose, which is then converted into glycogen, burned as fuel or stored as body fat. By itself, galactose is not found in nature, which makes sense because it works best with glucose.

  Galactose only breaks down in the liver; it doesn't shuttle itself into muscle glycogen as glucose does. For this reason, it's my humble opinion that when on a caloric surplus, galactose may be more prone to convert to fat gain than glucose, this is just a logical thought of mine.

When on a cut, muscle glycogen becomes even more important, so galactose seems very useless from a bodybuilding standpoint. Glucose clearly kicks galactoses ass in terms of simple sugars for the fitness fam. Galactose really shines when it becomes lactose, but we will go into that once we get to talking about disaccharides.

Please take into consideration that talking about this stuff is on a micro level, and while it's helpful, and gives you the edge to know, it's not going to make or break your diet. It's simply paving the way for you to understand the practical use of all the diets I will be breaking down in the next chapter.

• **Fructose** is seemingly the most demonized out of the 3 main simple sugars. But, to just call fructose deadly without any context is foolish. The main sources of fructose are fruits, fruit juice, honey, soft drinks sweetened by high-fructose corn syrup, and products sweetened by agave syrup or invert sugar.

We call fructose fruit sugar. This is because fruits are its main source, but fruits also contain other sugars, mostly glucose and sucrose. The problem isn't fructose itself, it's the isolated fructose in high dosages that's bad.

Just like galactose, fructose isn't really found in nature isolated in high quantities in any food.

In nature, fructose is normally with glucose making sucrose. Just as glucose and galactose make lactose.

When you have a 50/50 ratio of glucose and fructose in a meal, your body tends to do well absorbing all of it, even better when the ratio of glucose to fructose is higher, meaning less fructose and more glucose.

When fructose is consumed without glucose, and you're doing this often, you're creating problems for yourself. One of the biggest problems is that almost every cell in your body can use glucose, but only the liver can break down fructose which is fine in small dosages.

We have created refined versions, and isolated fructose, which by itself on high dosages is a huge burden on your liver. Your body is not designed to digest large amounts of fructose all of the time. I will tell you in a moment why isolated fructose even exists in the first place, but for now, let me explain to you why it's bad.

Firstly, it can hardly be burned as fuel when by itself so your body is trying to digest it, but not getting anything out of it. It's like a relationship between two people, you are your body, and fructose is your asshole boyfriend. But because you're putting all of the work into the relationship, and he is not giving you anything back, your body (you) is going downhill.

Since your body can't absorb large amounts of fructose well, bad things happen when we consume abnormally high amounts habitually, all while being sedentary most of the time. Welcome to America, my friend, or as I like to call it "MERCA". This had caused all kinds of problems like yours truly, "Diabetes".

Some people that are diagnosed with irritable bowel syndrome may actually just be eating too much shit. Pardon my French, you guys may just be eating to many refined foods containing isolated fructose in the form of HFCS.

Here are all of the fun things that the American diet high on refined sugars does for us, we get to enjoy: excessive abdominal bloating and gas (flatulence), abdominal cramps and pain, diarrhea, constipation, nausea, vomiting, excessive belching, heartburn (gastric reflux) and lethargy or depression within several hours of ingesting fructose.

One thing to note, and this a micro reason to the antidote of having a "balanced diet of fat/carb/protein", is that certain amino acids also help the body to absorb things like fructose. This is why we should never demonize a macronutrient, because they all work together like 3 CEO's of large, interconnected companies.

One last, really bad thing that happens with isolated fructose is that a larger amount of it is usually stored as fat than almost any other fuel source. Hopefully, this strikes an epiphany for you, "OMG" this is where the term "dirty carbs" came from! Wow, this is why simple sugars were demonized in the first place.

It's not that simple sugars are bad; it's the isolation of fructose and galactose that large food companies have taken advantage of for the sole purpose of increasing their profit margin. The reason that learning from TV, magazines or food companies is bad, is because all of these people are in it to sell to you. Their opinions are highly biased, and their advertising is nothing more than subliminal messaging to your cerebral cortex saying "buy me," "I'm good for you", or "I'm cool", or "I have a great story."

The truth is, in 1975, we introduced isolated fructose into just about everything as "high-fructose corn syrup," which become a multi-billion-dollar boom for the corn industry. HFCS was cheaper than any other sweetener and much sweeter than sucrose, which was what we used before. 1975 was when the economy rose, and the health of America dropped. This is when diabetes and heart disease started to become much more prominent.

This is also when many new medications were developed for diabetes, heart disease, and other illnesses causes by our newly refined diets. Basically, this was steroids for the economy: more profit in the processed food industry meant more jobs at mills and such. More people with illnesses meant more doctors, higher production of medicine, etc. The FDA let this pass. After all, the government, the U.S., the food industry, it's all one big business.

Oh, and we get to blame foods with fat for this

so we can then promote more refined shit. Fun fact, fructose also elevates triglycerides - animal fat? Eh, not so much. The truth of the matter is, if we were dumb enough to buy into an idea or be deceived then we deserved it. That's why people like me write books like this.

Let's end this little refined food war with a bang. Here are some things that isolated fructose can provide for you: cardiovascular disease, liver disease, cancer, arthritis, even gout and depletion of vitamins and minerals. But hey, don't hate fructose, just understand the evolution of food and how the economy ties into the increase of obesity.

The thing is, it's not all the economy's fault, it's 50% our fault as well, and I am giving you the knowledge, tools and firepower to do something about it. Onward, to disaccharides.

Double Carbs (Disaccharides)

These are the carbs that are midway in between simple carbs and complex carbs. Maybe we can just call them normal carbs or almost complex carbs. Basically, double carbs are two monosaccharides married together.

When a couple of single molecules meet, life happens, nature happens. When glucose and fructose sign paper documents to be bound together, they then become sucrose a/k/a table sugar. When galactose and glucose bump molecules, they become Lactose, which is that stuff in milk that scares us all shitless. And when two glucose molecules combine, we get Maltose, which you can find in most cereals, beer, and germinating seeds.

Let's look into these disaccharides independently to learn what we need to know about them.

- **Sucrose** is known as table sugar and table sugar is crystalized sucrose. Sucrose is made from glucose and fructose and occurs naturally in nature. Remember how I talked about fructose not being all bad? Well, in nature, fructose is always with glucose. When these are together making sucrose, your body has no trouble digesting these sugars.

  Fruits and vegetables contain fructose, so blankly saying fructose is bad as a statement is out of context. The synthesis and isolation of fructose is bad. When you consume fruits and vegetables, you're getting sucrose, so a nice mix of glucose and fructose as well as tons of vital vitamins and minerals that further help you digest the sugars and use them.

  Basically, sucrose is the sugar of nature, the richest edible sources comes from ripe dates, sugar beets, sweet peas, and most dried fruits. Sucrose shows up almost everywhere naturally in carb sources, including plants, vegetables and fresh fruits, which is why I am coining it "nature's sugar".

  While sucrose is still a sugar, it means going buck wild on sucrose habitually will be detrimental to your health. It's still much better for you than processed foods containing HFCS as the sweetener. When you're eating baked goods or processed foods (on occasion) "cough cough," read the ingredient lists, opt for products using sucrose as a sugar over HFCS. Your body will thank you in ten years.

- **Lactose** often gets bashed and has a bad name in the health industry. One of the biggest issues with lactose is that many individuals, especially from Asian and African countries, do not possess the enzyme lactase to properly digest this form of sugar.

  You can find lactose in milk, and across the board in dairy products such as cheese, yogurt, ice cream, butter, buttermilk and cream. Lactose is made up of 1 galactose molecule and 1 glucose molecule. For anyone that doesn't have an intolerance to lactose products, lactose normally also contains whey and casein protein. These two proteins mix well together which make products containing lactose good for bodybuilders, i.e. they help you build muscle.

  I digress, sorry, I am aware that I fall off topic a lot, but it's for your own understanding. Remember a little earlier when I was talking about how galactose shines when it becomes lactose, which happens when it combines with glucose? Yes? Ok, good. Let's think about this logically since we have both glucose and galactose working together. Galactose can run off to the liver and be converted into liver glucose and then burned for brain fuel and other fuel sources, while glucose shuttles into your muscles and becomes muscle glucose.

  The kicker is that lactose-containing foods typically have a great amino acid profile to help rebuild your muscles. See how carb and protein can work together here? One form of carb is fueling your brain and organs, while another is fueling your muscles, all while protein is being synthesized to rebuild your muscles bigger and stronger.

It's pretty cool how the body works on a micro level, you've got to love science. The point is, don't be afraid of dairy and lactose unless you have an intolerance. I am not saying to base your diet on lactose and dairy-containing products. I am just saying that they can have a place in your diet, they aren't always bad.

Anything can be considered bad in high amounts, in skewed contexts, and with individuals who may be intolerant to the substance. I am not telling you that anything is super bad or good, nor am I arguing from a biased position. I am simply telling you the facts in a practical fashion.

If your body is deficient in lactase, or does not produce it, then you should stay away from lactose and dairy. But if not, enjoy your dairy products with lactose sugar. If you're having symptoms like diarrhea, bloating, gas, etc., then make sure to check for different intolerances like fructose intolerance, gluten intolerance, or lactose intolerance.

It could even be many other things. Why is this important to someone reading a dieting and nutrition book who wants to build a badass physique? Well, I can tell you from experience, when you eat things that don't react well with your body, you don't perform well in the gym.

Sometimes you don't even have the motivation to go at all because you feel lethargic and tired. Not only that, if you're trying to get jacked and shredded, you don't want to be super bloated all the time, that doesn't look good.

Eating foods you have an intolerance to is even bad for muscle gain and fat loss because your body is going to be spending all of its energy trying to get rid of the food that it's struggling to digest. We want to look good, feel good, and perform optimally. To do so we need to be digesting as close to 100% of the food we eat as possible.

- **Maltose** is composed of 2 glucose molecules. Maltose is known as malt sugar. Since it's mainly found in cereal, beer, and germination seeds, it isn't a major part of most peoples' diets.

Ok, don't go and start drinking more beer with the justification of "I need more maltose." I will not be held accountable for you telling yourself you need more beer to fuel the muscle because Jordan Miller said so. This is exactly why having context in an argument or statement is crucial.

Maltose is an interesting sugar because of its use in alcohol. This process is called fermentation. Glucose, maltose and other sugars are converted to ethanol by yeast cells in the absence of oxygen. Maltose is uncommon in nature but it can be formed through the breakdown of starch by the enzymes of the mouth.

Maltose is much more boring in comparison to the controversy over sucrose and lactose, but nonetheless, it is one of the 3 main disaccharides that you ought to at least know about when understanding dieting. The reason I am going into all of this is so when we get to talking about actual diets and breaking them down, you will understand them on a molecular level.

- **Complex Carbs** should probably be known as the savior carbs, as we call them the almighty "clean carbs." But I just call them polysaccharides. These carbs have several chains of molecules. There are 3 main complex carbs that make up polysaccharides: Starch, Fiber, and Glycogen. These carbs are a little more complex, no pun intended, so we will go into each of them thoroughly.

- **Starch** is a complex carbohydrate, and is formed from long chains of glucose molecules. Here are the foods you will find high in starch: bread, grains, pasta, rice, cereal, potatoes, and beans. Getting rid of complex carbohydrates from the diet completely is a very bad idea.

Why do you think the diabetes and obesity rate is so high in America? Yep, we need to do better. Complex carbs provide the most sustainable source of energy out of any source of carbs. Complex carbs should be a staple in your diet for both building muscle and burning fat. Here is a long list you can use to map out your diet. These are the healthy complex carbs that contain starch. I have also listed some refined forms that you should stay away from.

(Whole Grains)

- Barley
- Oats
- Brown rice
- Quinoa (pronounced "keen'-wa")
- Buckwheat
- Rye
- Bulgur (cracked wheat)
- Triticale
- Couscous (refined wheat)
- Wheat berries
- Wild rice

(Unrefined Flours)

- Barley
- Rice
- Buckwheat
- Rye
- Soy
- Garbanzo beans
- Triticale
- Lima bean
- Wheat
- Oat
- Whole wheat pastry

- Potato

(Egg-Free Pastas)

Pastas come in many shapes including spaghetti, macaroni, lasagna noodles, flat noodles, spirals, wheels, alphabet noodles, etc. Most of these are made from highly refined flours and therefore should play a small role in your diet.

- Artichoke pasta

- Tomato pasta

- Corn pasta (no wheat)

- Whole wheat pasta

- Spinach pasta

- Rice pasta (no wheat)

(Asian Noodles) Most of these are made from highly refined flours and therefore should play a small role in your diet.

- Bean threads

- Somen

- Buckwheat soba

- Udon

- Rice noodles

(Roots)

- Burdock

- Sweet potatoes

- Celeriac (celery root)

- Tapioca
- Jerusalem artichoke (sunchoke)
- Taro root
- Jicama
- Water chestnuts
- Parsnips
- White potatoes
- Rutabaga
- Yams

(Winter Squashes)

- Butternut
- Acorn
- Hubbard
- Banana
- Pumpkin
- Buttercup
- Turban squash
- Legumes

(Beans)

- Aduki (Azuki)
- Red kidney
- Black
- Mung

- Fava (broad)
- Navy
- Garbanzo (chick-peas)
- Pink
- Great northern
- Pinto
- Limas
- White kidney (cannellini)

(Lentils)

- Brown
- Red
- Green

(Peas)

- Black-eyed
- Split yellow
- Split green
- Whole green

Starchy carbs should make up a large portion of your diet. These carbs are high in nutrients, are much better for regulating your blood sugar, and keep you feeling full and healthy. When you feel satiated you don't need to eat as much to fulfill your hunger needs, which equates to less overall caloric intake, by nature.

Your health, no matter how shredded you are and

how jacked you are, is not solely predicated on how many complex carbs you eat, but it definitely plays a role in performance, mood, building muscle, burning fat and overall health.

- **Fiber** is a carbohydrate that many people think is actually a vitamin or a mineral. Fiber is like the secret spy carb that cleanses your colon of its sins. Fiber is a very valuable nutrient that most of the world is deficient in. Fiber can't be digested; it's resistant to the digestive enzymes in the human body.

  You will find fiber in fruits, vegetables, legumes, grains, and nuts. Consuming enough fiber is crucial in helping to prevent things like colon cancer, diabetes and cardiovascular disease. It even has a positive effect on lowering LDL cholesterol. There are 2 main types of fiber: insoluble fiber and soluble fiber.

  Insoluble fiber speeds up GI transit, slows down starch hydrolysis, increases fecal weight, and delays glucose absorption.

  Soluble fiber delays GI transport, lowers blood cholesterol (LDL), and delays glucose absorption, all very important stuff.

  Fiber is even more complex than that: insoluble fiber comes in 3 different forms as does soluble fiber. I know you're probably wondering what the different sub categories of fiber have to do with getting jacked and shredded, but think about it from an artistic standpoint.

  Your body is your canvas and nutrients are your

artistry tools. Your long-term results are predicated on your level of knowledge and application of nutrition, which make up 75% of your jacked and shredded results. Different fibers play different specific roles in nutrient digestion.

If you want to build muscle and get lean blood sugar regulation, then proper digestion is a key factor. Having a strong, powerful, lean body means being healthy.

- **Cellulose** is a form of insoluble fiber which you will find in fruits, vegetables and legumes. The crazy thing about cellulose as a fiber, and as a polysaccharide, is the fact that it's found in wood and cotton.

Cellulose is also the most abundant polymer on planet earth. In case you don't know what a polymer is, polymer is just another name for a large molecule, i.e. a macromolecule. Macromolecules make up macronutrients.

Cotton is actually 90% cellulose fiber, and wood is 40-50% cellulose fiber. We are even experimenting with the use of cellulose as biofuel. Cellulose in big business is mainly used to make paper. But can we eat paper, wood, cotton and biofuel? We can't eat cotton because we can't digest that much cellulose.

Actually, we can't digest it at all, and it's toxic to us. Raw cotton has something called gossypol inside it, which will damage our liver and heart.

Basically, eating cotton will kill you slowly, unless you have four stomachs and make moo sounds. Wood isn't edible either, still way too much fiber for us to try and breakdown. The amount of fiber in wood and cotton is way higher than edible food so we can't handle it.

Although scientists are working on different types of edible wood; yes, edible wood is a thing, just not in nature. One day you may be fitting Yacaratia wood into your macros, but for now, it's only served as a delicious dessert in Argentina.

Paper is nothing more than refined wood so don't try and eat it. I highly doubt we will ever make edible paper in America, maybe in some 3rd world countries.

On to the point of why I am telling you this, we often argue about health in terms of, "Is it natural or manmade?" This is actually an irrational argument because both manmade foods and organic foods can be toxic. Just because something is organic, doesn't mean it's good for you, and just because something is refined doesn't mean it's really bad.

It comes down to chemicals, and chemical reactions in the body - chemistry. When you isolate whey protein, i.e. refine certain protein molecules from dairy, it creates a very healthy refined food known as a protein shake or protein powder. In the same token, if you isolate fructose from glucose, or refine it, which also doesn't happen in nature, it slowly kills your liver and is basically toxic when consumed habitually.

We need fiber in our diet to keep us healthy and to help us perform optimally as athletes, and fiber is in cotton, so logically organic cotton should help us? Nope. Yes, cotton and wood are natural and contain the same types of fibers that are in fruits and vegetables, but our bodies can't digest them.

The point of what I am saying, is that how healthy something is can't be solely predicated on how refined or organic the food is. It depends upon the chemical and molecular structure of the food. Some processed food is healthier than some organic options and vice versa. We are still learning about what is edible, and what is optimal for muscle growth and fat loss. But I want you to understand two things right now.

You need to be open minded when it comes to this stuff, and you need to ask questions, don't just assume that something is good or bad because of some bullshit scientific study. Make that decision yourself, but make it in a well-educated and safe manner.

I digress, cellulose is everywhere, and it's actually the main building material of the cells of plants.

The name cellulose actually became the name of this fiber because of the way it was discovered. Cellulose was first isolated in 1834 by French chemist Anselme Payen. He obtained the new substance from the "cell" walls of plants. This lead to him appropriately coining this fiber as "Cellulose".

Ever since its discovery, we've known that since we can't digest cellulose, it passes through our system un-broken down. It internally acts as a roughage that helps the movements of our intestines. That effect is what helps us dodge colon cancer.

· **Hemicelluloses** Before I go into this, let me state that there is both insoluble hemicelluloses and soluble hemicelluloses fiber. I know it's tricky and I have to try and avoid a hemi headache, too. You may be wondering, what is the molecular difference between hemicelluloses and cellulose? The difference is that cellulose is made up of thousands of long chains of glucose, while hemicellulose can be made up of different monosaccharides.

Hemicelluloses, just like cellulose, helps in the digestion of food, helps regulate blood sugar, and for a combination of many different reasons why I won't go into, helps with weight loss. This is not a chemistry encyclopedia so I am going to try to keep from going too crazy on the small nuances of molecules. You can find your insoluble hemicellulose in celery and lettuce and your soluble versions in rolled oats and oat bran.

· **Lignin** is an insoluble fiber that is mostly found in flaxseed, carrots, and strawberries. It is present in all vascular plants and helps to make vegetables firm and crunchy. Lignin, like cellulose, is one of the most abundant polymers on planet earth, however cellulose is still king.

Lignin is good for heart health and even possibly, the immune system. P.S we're still not sure about its relation to immune function, so do not quote me on that, because I am not giving you any BS study saying "it may" be good for immune function.

- **Pectin** is a soluble fiber naturally found in citrus fruits, vegetables, and apples. Pectin slows the passage of food through the GI tract and helps to lower blood cholesterol. It is also known to regulate stool size and stop diarrhea.

    Pectin has also been shown to reduce heartburn by reducing the amount of food and acid concentration reaching the esophagus. Here are the studies conducted using pectin for heartburn relief:

40. Waterhouse ET, Washington C, Washington N. An investigation into the efficacy of the pectin based anti-reflux formulation-Aflurax. Int J Pharm. 2000;209(1-2):79-85.

41. Havelund T, Aalykke C. The efficacy of a pectin-based raft-forming anti-reflux agent in endoscopy-negative reflux disease. (Scand J Gastroenterol. 1997;32(8):773-777.

42. Kapadia CJ, Mane VB. Raft-forming agents: antireflux formulations. Drug Dev Ind Pharm. 2007;33(12):1350-1361).

Why is this important as a physique builder? Do you know how easy it is to get heartburn and consistently be blowing up the bathroom because of some pre-workout and mass gainer you decided to try? It happens, and if it hasn't happened to you yet, be ready for it to happen.

If you're getting heartburn or indigestion, your body is not taking full advantage of the fuel you're feeding it, which means a lot of those amino acids and carbohydrates that could be used to build muscle are going to waste. Diarrhea is pretty much the quickest way to become dehydrated. You can't do shit, nada, nothing regarding performance in the gym after the dehydration of diarrhea.

Heartburn and diarrhea together will absolutely kill your gains, happiness, butthole, and life, so do you think it's important to know which foods have pectin and when this fiber may be of help to you?

You need to be getting this fiber so that your body can focus on things you want to happen, like the building of lean body mass and not the burden of trying to get rid of the acid trying to kill your esophagus like WW3 and diarrhea trying to rip your soul out of your anus. If you are trying to make gains, you need to avoid indigestion and diarrhea like the plague, end of correlation.

- **Gums/Mucilage** is the oddball soluble fiber. You can find it in guar gum, carrageenan and gum arabic. All you really need to know is that these fibers slow the passage of food through the gastrointestinal tract and help lower blood cholesterol. Better cholesterol, better digestion, it's not a game.

Now there are many more minute forms of fiber out there but these are the main forms of fiber. These are the forms of fiber that are most valuable to know about and understand.

Why for muscle building?

I know I have already mentioned this many times, but I need to scientifically iron it onto your head. **Carbohydrates are well known to be protein sparing**.

This means that carbohydrates give protein a red carpet pathway to building muscle. Carbs protect the protein you consume from being converted to glucose to serve as an energy source when glycogen and plasma glucose levels decrease.

This is known as gluconeogenesis. This happens when blood glucose concentrations become too low, which in turn causes the release of the hormone glucagon. You don't want this, avoid this like you avoided telling anyone about what you did at that party a couple of years ago. Just like all of the alcohol puts your brain in a potential position of losing, this gluconoblablacornpuffs stuff puts your muscles in the position to lose.

This is where you become catabolic or muscle wasting. You probably want to avoid this just like you avoided that pizza at Planet Fitness, unless you enjoy losing muscle, gaining fat, decreasing your metabolism and losing strength.

Carbs also fuel the brain; glucose is the brain's main source of fuel. Carbs are very important for the proper functioning of your central nervous system (CNS). Just so you know, your CNS is what allows your brain to send electrical impulses to your muscles to tell them to contract, and allows them to learn motor patterns such as bench press, squat and deadlift.

Your CNS is absolutely the biggest factor in gaining strength besides building muscle. The stronger the CNS, the better adaptations you will make to exercise; the better your adaptations to certain exercises, the more strength you gain on them.

The more strength you gain on compound movements, the more muscle you will be set up to build; the more muscle you build, the faster your metabolism expends calories. In other words, a healthy CNS means a bigger, leaner and stronger physique.

Low carbs will also wake up an evil beast called hypoglycemia (or low blood sugar) that kills your energy. Symptoms include, obviously, hunger, dizziness, weakness and fatigue. Nothing will destroy your strength and eat your muscle like a nice walk in the park with hypoglycemia.

Carbclusion

Like how I did that? So, now that you understand carbs, the ins and the outs and how most of it will play a role in your health and the building of your physique, where do we go from here? Don't worry, my impressionable friend, in the chapters to come we will cover everything, and I do mean "EVERYTHING."

We will go over the ratios of macronutrients that may work best for you, as well as what type of dieting methods/ eating plans may work best for you, depending on tons of different factors. But first we need to talk about protein and carbs so please, take a break from this book and let this knowledge about carbs sink in. This journey you are embarking upon? It's not an antidote, it's a marathon; a journey and a lifestyle, so please don't rush through this book.

PROTEIN

While most sedentary people consume enough protein, a lot of people looking to live a healthy active lifestyle don't. When working out with weights, becoming more active, burning fat and building muscle, you will need much more protein than the normal sedentary person.

The USDA recommends 10% - 35% of your diet come from protein. If you're reading this book and looking to learn how to get lean and build muscle, you will be towards the higher point of protein. Instead of looking at percentages for protein, I like to use bodyweight. .8 – 1.2 grams of protein per pound of bodyweight is a good number to shoot for. Taking that range into account, the amount of protein you should use per pound of bodyweight should be based off of your body fat, age, gender, body type, and goals.

Protein is the macronutrient building block that your body uses to rebuild itself. Let's break this down; these are the things protein does for you:

- Growth (this is especially important for children, teens, and pregnant women).

- Protein is the macronutrient responsible for all tissue repair.
- Protein is crucial to build a strong immune system.
- Protein is important for taking care of your hormones and enzymes.
- Your body converts protein into energy when carbohydrates aren't available.
- Preserving and building of lean muscle mass.

These are the food items that you can look to for your protein consumption in order to meet your daily protein goals: meats, poultry, fish, meat substitutes, cheese, milk, nuts, legumes, and in smaller quantities, in starchy foods and vegetables.

When we eat protein sources such as meat, fish and poultry, our body breaks down the protein that they contain into amino acids (the building blocks of protein). Some of these amino acids are essential, meaning that we need to get them from our diet, and other are nonessential, which means that our body can make them itself.

Luckily for us, the protein that comes from animal sources contains all of the essential amino acids that we need. The thing is, plant sources are much more difficult to extract the essential amino acids from. If you are on a plant based diet, getting protein is a little more difficult but none the less doable.

Top 5 Bang for Your Buck Proteins

There are tons of different sources of protein out there, all with different amino acid profiles and different levels of bio-available protein. The quality of protein is measured by Biological Value (BV). "But Jordan, what does *that* mean"? BV is the value that measures how well the body can absorb and utilize a protein. The higher the BV, the more your body can absorb, use and retain the protein you're consuming.

What this means for you is that the protein with the highest BV gives you the best bang for your buck regarding "GAINZ". The famous "whey protein" has the highest BV value of any source of protein at 104. Egg protein comes in second place with a BV of 100. Milk protein comes in a close third with a strong value of 91, which is still "A" grade protein in my book!

Beef has a BV rating of around 80 putting it in 4th place, and soy protein comes in losing the fight at a rating of 74 of the BV scale. Here is a little chart showing the different BV levels from high too low.

Whey - *104-159*
Egg - *100*
Cow's Milk - *91*
Casein - *80*
Soy - *74*
Beef - *80*
Fish - *83*
Chicken - *79*
Wheat Gluten - *54*
Kidney Beans – *49*

1. **Whey Protein,** as crazy as it sounds, was once a byproduct that was once thrown away by dairy manufacturers. Now whey protein is the pinnacle of sports nutrition supplements. Whey protein is the highest BV source of protein, period. It's not

only the highest BV protein, but it also enters the blood stream the fastest.

Whey protein is also the highest in BCAAs (Branched Chain Amino Acids), as well as glutamine. Whey is known as the anabolic protein since it increases protein synthesis so much over other protein sources.

Here's the fun part, you must be educated: there are 3 different types of whey protein supplements on the market: whey protein concentrate, whey protein isolate and whey hydroslate.

The concentrated version of whey is normally between 50-80 percent protein. The isolate separates whey from lactose, ash, fats and carbs so that you can receive 90-97 percent protein.

Then you have your micro filtered whey isolate. Whey hydroslate is the most expensive protein you can get your hands on, if you have a fetish for spending money on protein. This stuff had already digested into peptides before it hits your stomach, so this means it will go straight into your bloodstream after taking it.

Want to know my opinion on whey protein? Well, I am going to tell you whether you want to know or not. I don't take whey protein as a supplement. Now, this is a personal preference, I work from home so the convenience of protein in a shake isn't a big thing for me.

I think whey protein is awesome but is the amount of money you spend on the super high tech hydroslate worth it? In my humble opinion, hell no, are you kidding me? Spending $80 on a jug of protein does not appease me. The price difference from concentrate to hydro does not justify the subsequent amount of difference in results.

I am a firm believer that whey protein is not a must. It does make a difference, a very small difference, on a micro level. While it's important to understand bio availability and the rate of digestion of a diverse range of proteins, you can't take it to heart.

I personally stick to eggs and chicken for my main sources of protein, although technically whey protein is superior.

If you're eating enough protein throughout your day, I would not stress it. If you're eating high BV sources of protein like eggs, chicken, beef, diary, milk, etc. and getting in at least your bodyweight in protein, you should be good. Think of whey protein as a tool in your arsenal. You need quick, high quality protein? Whey is your best friend in that case.

Sometimes we miss meals, sometimes we don't hit our protein macros for the day, and we are all busy sometimes. In the case of being busy or without a protein source, do yourself a favor and grab a protein shake or bar. Some people enjoy protein shakes and bars, they have become much tastier lately, this is for certain.

Honestly, I am a big fan of protein cookies. If you haven't tried protein cookies yet and you like cookies, then you are missing out. Because of all the research and the scientific conclusion about whey protein, we now have tons of whey protein infused foods. Whey protein infused peanut butter, bread, cookies, pancakes, brownies, cereals, chips, etc. You name it, there is probably a high protein version infused with whey protein.

This whole protein infusion trend has caused a big stir between the all-natural crowd and the fitness crowd. In my opinion, you don't need these protein-infused products, but they can definitely make dieting and hitting macros much more fun.

I think protein infused things are a beautiful thing. Granted, I really don't like products with high amounts of high fructose corn syrup so watch out for HFCS no matter what the product is.

At the end of the day, whey protein is awesome but it all comes down to how much money you are willing to spend. I recommend if you're on a budget and looking for a protein supplement, to just go to your local Wal-Mart and grab some $20 whey concentrate. In terms of bang for your buck, you can't beat that $20 Wal-Mart protein.

When you want to step up to a higher grade, personally my two favorite protein companies are Optimum Nutrition and MTS. MTS whey protein is arguably the best tasting protein in the world. We need to understand whey protein for exactly what it is: a convenient and versatile source of super high quality, muscle building protein, end of story.

2. **Egg Protein** is one of the cheapest and most

versatile forms of protein out there, hopefully you are already eating eggs. Let me start by saying one whole egg contains 6 grams of high quality protein. This protein is so good that it's used as a gold standard to measure other foods as protein sources.

Eggs are also a very rich source of vitamins such as A, E and K, as well as a range of B vitamins like B12, riboflavin and folic acid. That's not even the best part; eggs contain all 8 essential amino acids needed for optimal muscle recovery and building minerals like calcium, zinc and iron. I know you're probably wondering, "what about the 5 grams of fat?"

Here's the thing: first of all, this fat is very healthy fat, so don't believe anyone who says that eggs are bad for you. A couple of egg yolks a day are very healthy. When you're eating a whole egg you have 5 grams of fat, and 6 grams of protein.

If you are trying to come up with a high protein meal, I recommend opting for 1-2 whole eggs and to get the rest of your protein in the meal from egg whites. One egg white is 3 to 3.5 grams of protein. If you are looking to get 30 grams of protein in your meal and about 10 grams of healthy fat, use 2 whole eggs, which will get us to 12 grams of protein. Now add 5 egg whites to the mix to get your total of 30 grams of protein. Now you have a great fat/protein balanced meal with current macros of 10 Fat and 30 protein.

Now add a piece of fruit and a complex carb and you have yourself a nice balanced meal. Think of eggs as a great template for a high protein meal. Tailor the amount of egg yolks and egg whites to meet your protein goals for the day. Want to build a physique? You will need to get used to doing a little basic math on a daily basis. Lots of fun. But it becomes really easy and second nature after you have played 'build a diet' for a couple of months.

3. **Milk Protein** is just like egg protein, not really, but it's another great source of high quality protein to support your selfish addiction to making "GAINZ". Milk protein is made up of some whey protein but mostly casein protein.

The mix of these two proteins gives it a unique blend of mostly slow, and some faster digesting proteins, since milk is made up of 80% casein protein and 20% whey. One of the things that casein does that's different from whey is that it releases into the bloodstream much more slowly. Casein is a slow burning source of protein. Milk contains good fats, good carbs, and extremely high quality whey and casein protein. This makes milk nature's protein drink.

Before we had whey protein shakes, bodybuilders and powerlifters chugged milk all of the time as well as mixed in eggs for a high quality protein cocktail. Fortunately, we have protein shakes now, which is just another way of doing this.

The thing is, now our protein cocktails taste damn good. We are living in the golden age of fitness. Some of us are just not educated enough to realize it. With all of the macronutrient data you are reading in this book, you should understand how a natural drink with good fats, good carbs, and high quality protein is extremely vital to your "GAINZ". You want to look for these high quality sources of protein for making strength, power and muscle gains as well as getting shredded.

I know you will probably hear contradictory statements about all of the things I am talking about on TV and the Internet. Make sure you pay attention to the context of these highly biased statements before you try and take them for any practical value in your life. What I mean by this is that some people will say eggs are bad for you, milk is not for humans, blah blah blah.

You can say anything is good or bad for you depending on the context of your statement. Be careful: going back and forth, getting confused, and then getting stressed is the reason most people say it's not worth it.

The truth is, it's not complicated, but everyone has their own opinion about what is healthy, and what you should do. This is not for anyone else to decide, just you. I am not telling you what you must do, I am presenting you with the facts and the unbiased, unmolested info that will be most practical for you.

I promise this stuff is not stressful; it's fun when you're winning at this fitness game, and after you read this book YOU WILL BE WINNING. If this book doesn't open your eyes and change your life, return it, because I am not here to waste your time or money. I don't want your money, I want to see you WIN at health and fitness.

4. **You Got Beef?** If not, you should think about trying beef for a strong source of protein. Beef protein, like casein protein, provides you with a slow releasing protein. Slow releasing proteins will keep you feeling fuller longer, and also will keep you making "DEM GAINZ."

   Beef protein is also super abundant in blood building iron as well as B-vitamins. These are things that contribute to nutrient utilization + energy production. Beef protein is digested in the stomach, which means when you are eating beef, it won't cause that slight bloat in your intestines that whey protein causes from intestinal digestion.

   This is helpful to know when doing things such a photo shoots. You want to think about looking for slower digesting proteins that don't bloat your intestines, so when getting ready for physique shots, opt for non-bloating foods and non-bloating protein sources like beef.

   When looking for sources of beef, look for lean beef, the leaner the better. Try to at least go for 80/20 lean beef. If you are trying to get lean and are in prep for a contest or photoshoot, opt for something like 97/3 lean beef. Beware, beef of that caliber is very pricey - you pay to play my friend. The fitness game is always give and take, it's all about balance.

5. **Casein** protein is the star child of milk and many other dairy products. Whey is a fast digesting

protein that results in rapid increase in blood amino acids, as well as protein synthesis. Casein, on the contrary, boasts a prolonged increase in blood amino acids that result in 34% reduction in protein breakdown.

So, by nature casein is a slower burning protein, and whey is a faster burning protein. With that said, having both casein and whey in your daily diet is a great way to ensure you're feeding your muscles 24/7. Having a mix of casein and whey in the diet will help slow protein breakdown and also ensure that your body is using the protein to rebuild, and not burning it as fuel.

I am not going bro here, I am not telling you that you should become a bro artist with your whey protein and casein protein, let me clarify. There are bullshit myths that you need to consume whey protein first thing in the morning and first thing after you work out or you will go "catabolic." This is simply not the case. It doesn't work that way.

Anabolism vs. catabolism comes down to a few simple factors. If you are on a caloric surplus, you can't be catabolic as long as you're hitting your protein numbers for the day. If you eat 150 grams of protein a day, it doesn't make a difference whether those meals are during your breakfast and post workout or not.

Personally, I haven't had a post workout protein shake or a breakfast shake in over a year, and I have built more muscle this past year than I have in the past 2 years. Why, you ask? Because I have been much more consistently in a caloric surplus day in and day out over this past year. The two years prior I would dip into a caloric deficit more often because I was more focused on staying lean than getting big.

When you're on a caloric deficit for a prolonged period of time you will be a little catabolic, but timing your protein for breakfast and post workout won't change that. The best way to ensure minimal muscle loss or to stop it, is to lose the weight very slowly, one pound a week is my preferred rate.

This is also highly dependent on the body fat level you are starting out at, as well as your end goal and deadline. We will go more into this in part four. The reason that casein and whey should be known and understood is because of a couple things.

Whey protein is a higher quality protein but it burns more quickly, so without a mix of other proteins, you're not giving your body any slower burning proteins. Casein, on the other hand, burns much, much more slowly. It's my personal opinion that having both in your diet will result in stronger gains overtime, as well as better health. The thing is we know that slow digesting foods are crucial for regulating blood pressure, digestion, satiety and many other things.

We also know that foods that digest much more quickly, like foods containing simple sugars and easily digestible proteins, are very high in quality regarding vitamins, minerals, important amino acids and the body's preferred sources of readily burnable fuels.

In conclusion, having a mix of different types of protein would be much more valuable to you in the long run than sticking to just whey, or just casein. The slower digesting proteins allow the higher digesting proteins to be used 100% as building blocks, not as fuel. This is why milk is freaking awesome as well as all other dairy products! Eat your dairy for gains, unless you have a lactose intolerance.

Amino Acids

When you eat protein, your body breaks it down into the building blocks which are called "Amino Acids."

Why am I going into depth about the breakdown of proteins, you may ask? Well, if you understand protein and how it breaks down from a micro standpoint, it will be much easier to decipher which information in blog posts and magazine articles are relevant, and which articles are marketing shenanigans with no real world, educational value.

Anybody can tell you to do something a certain way, I am not doing that, I am giving you the facts without the biased marketing BS. Back to the topic, when protein is broken down in the body, a split happens; the protein splits into amino acids that all go and do separate jobs.

It's kind of like the Justice League broke apart in order to go do the unique things they're especially good at. All of their jobs are super important. This is why understanding the job of each amino acid is important – it helps you understand how each amino acid is very helpful for reaching specific goals, such as muscle building.

There are about 20-22 amino acids, 8 of which are

considered 'essential', which means your body can't make them. Since our bodies aren't able to synthesize them, we must consume them in food. If we don't consume them in food, the world will end. Kidding, but the point is, we need them, especially if we want to build a respectable physique.

The Super Essential 8

1. **Histidine** This amino acid is responsible for the growth and repair of tissues of all kinds, all *kindz* of gains, like white blood cell gains - you want white blood cell gains! Now let me blow your mind real quick. Histidine is important for nerve health in preventing unintended impulses that can lead to serious defects in the brain and spinal cord.

   That means this amino acid helps your body send signals to your brain and keeps your spine in working order. It even has a manufacturing firm named Histidinory that builds little white blood cells. If you didn't catch that, it was a joke. Your body doesn't actually have manufacturing firms, silly rabbit, lucky charms are for kids. Just making sure you're awake so you don't miss the next two paragraphs!

   Histidine even helps with radiation protection and aids in the removal of excess metals (like iron) from the body. This amino acid also produces gastric juices in the stomach that help speed up and improve digestion.

   However, the most intriguing thing about this amino acid is that it may aid in longer orgasms and better sexual enjoyment if you are um, having trouble in that area... So ladies and gentlemen, for longer lasting orgasms and more white blood cells, get in your Histidine. (Sources: dairy, meat, poultry, fish as well as rice, wheat and rye.)

2. **Lysine** This amino acid is very important for growth and development. Your body uses this amino acid for calcium absorption. You want calcium absorption because it results in bone and muscle growth as well as the conversion of fat into energy, yes that means fat burning.

Lysine also helps to maintain lean body mass in periods of extreme stress and fatigue. Here is why you care about this amino acid in terms of making gains: it is needed to produce antibodies, hormones (GH, testosterone, insulin, and more), enzymes, and collagen to repair damaged tissue, just like Histidine and many other essential amino acids.

Lysine helps in the building of new muscle protein, so this amino acid does aid in the building of new muscle as well as the maintenance of muscle when cutting weight. Lastly, it helps maintain healthy blood vessels which equals better blood flow. This is where you can get your precious Lysine: all dairy products, almonds, avocados, nuts, and seeds.

3. **Phenylalanine** This amino acid elevates the mood by stimulating the central nervous system, and may be important for motivation for whatever you need to be motivated for. This amino acid is secretly Tony Robbins. If you don't know Tony

Robbins, Google him to understand his relevance. Tony Robbins increases levels of epinephrine, nor-epinephrine, and dopamine in the anterior pituitary.

All three of these are neurotransmitters needed for peak performance of the nervous system. It also helps you to absorb UV rays from sunlight. This in turn gives a higher rate of Vitamin D, a strong hormone that you probably didn't know was a hormone.

A lot of the time this amino acid gets a bad rap because of skewed info in the media. Phenylalanine is used as a non-carbohydrate sweetener in any pop/soda/soft drink (combined with aspartic acid, as aspartame). Aspartame is simply the combination of the non-essential amino acid (Aspartic Acid) and the essential amino acid Phenylalanine, with a small amount of Methanol added to the mix. The thing is, there is more methanol in orange juice than diet soft drinks.

Thinking a little bit of aspartame is going to hurt you is dumb, and there are no studies to back these ignorant claims, just don't binge drink 2 liter bottles of diet soft drinks and you won't OD on aspartame... Water would probably kill you just as quickly as diet soda; on high dosages, anything is dangerous.

Aspartame being really bad is simply hippy bullshit. I digress, let's get back to Phenylalanine. Don't take his supplement if you are a pregnant woman or are diabetic. It results in higher blood pressure, headaches, nausea, heart trouble and nerve damage. If you don't have any health issues and you're not a pregnant woman, your golden, pony boy.

Here are some natural places to find this amino acid: all dairy products, almonds, avocados, nuts, and seeds. In terms of getting jacked and shredded, this amino acid allows maximal muscle contraction and relaxation. This means more gains and better recovery to tickle your fancy.

4. **Meth** Actually, Methionine is the name of the amino acid at hand, but I thought I'd give it a cute nickname. Anyways, this guy's main job is the breakdown of fats. Better break down of fats = higher testosterone rates. Higher testosterone = more gains, let's get jacked, "bro," and let's get jacked with that meth. Meth is a precursor to cysteine, which is the amino that produces glutathione to detoxify the liver.

   It's one of the three amines that are needed to manufacture creatine monohydrate within the body. Here is where you can find meth: Meat, fish, beans, eggs, garlic, lentils, onions, yogurt and seeds.

Creatine

Creatine or ATP (adenosine triphosphate) is a nitrogenous organic acid that helps to supply energy to all cells in the body, primary muscle cells.

The human body is made up of approximately 1% creatine. Out of that 1%, 0.14% is in the brain, 0.50% is in the muscle, and 0.18 is in the testes. The tiny amount left over is located in the liver, kidneys and other parts of the body.

Creatine is naturally found in food, especially high-grade beef and creatine supplements are very popular in the sports and nutrition world. It is used by athletes, bodybuilders, wrestlers, sprinters - just about anyone who is looking to gain muscle mass.

Creatine is scientifically proven to help you build muscle, but the thing is, it only gives you about a 1% boost in building muscle. Still, it's one of the only supplements scientifically proven to improve muscle hypertrophy with long-term supplementation.

Since your muscles use creatine as a primary source of fuel, it only makes sense that giving them a little more than the body produces gives you a 1% edge. Do you need supplement with creatine? No, but it's a great option to look into after you have been lifting for 3-5 years.

I recommend around 5 grams a day for the average-sized male looking to get that 1% edge, I am talking to you, the guy who is on the fence about creatine. Yes, it works, but the effect is so small you will never notice or feel it. Just know in the back of your mind that it helps you just a tiny, tiny bit if you decide to take it.

For women smaller than 130lbs, I recommend 2-3 grams a day for supplementation. For giants, I recommend 6-8 grams a day - you know who you are, you 300lb mountain Viking mutha F**ka.

For your mom I recommend, stop I'm kidding bro, bye Felicia, I digress.

If you have kidney problems stay away from creatine; it doesn't end well for people with kidney problems. No need to cycle completely off creatine, just cycle down to a lower dosage and purge at high dosages. If you start at

5 grams, cycle down to 3 for a couple months from time to time. If you start at 2-3, cycle down to 1-2 every couple months, and if you're starting at 6-8, cycle down to 4-5 from time to time.

That's all folks, creatine is natural and safe for the most part and it may already be in your pre-workout anyways. P.S. read your labels, cot damnit! That's it, that's all you need to know about creatine, it is what it is.

BCAA'S

Branched chain amino acids (BCAA'S) are 3 amino acids that are widely regarded as the "bodybuilding amino acids." BCAA'S are the most important amino acids when it comes to manufacturing, maintaining and repairing muscle-tissue.

There are three BCAA'S: Leucine, Iso-leucine, and Valine. They have little anabolic affect by themselves. However, you put them together in the right doses and you have yourself ANABOLIC STERIODS. I'm kidding, BCAA's aren't steroids, although high school boys think BCAA's (and creatine, for that matter) are steroids.

It is believed that a 2-1-2 equilibrium in Leucine/Iso-leucine/Valine dosing yields the best results. The dosages listed are the FDA recommendations for taking the individual BCAA's.

BCAA's are even used to treat depression. Protein deficiencies are a legitimate concern for most of the world because the FDA recommends your protein intake be 10% of your body's daily calories at the low set point, and 35% at the high set point.

But how does that help anybody? Just to make life easier, base your protein off of your lean body mass and bodyweight, not a percentage of your daily calories. Your protein intake should be tailored to you. BCAA's are a popular supplement for weightlifters and bodybuilders, but in the grand scheme of things they are still just that "a supplement."

The point of BCAA's is to "supplement" an already capable diet. If your diet is in check and you can afford to try BCAA's in supplement form without hurting your wallet, go for it. But remember, supplements are only going to make that 1% difference. *Your daily diet and physical activity is what will produce 99% of your results.* Let's get back to the three BCAA's:

1. **Leucine** This amino acid is the strongest of the BCAA's and it's responsible for the regulation of blood-sugar levels, the growth and repair of tissue, skin, bones and, of course, skeletal muscle. Leucine is a strong potentiator to Human Growth Hormone (HGH). It helps in healing wounds, regulating energy, and assists in preventing the breakdown of muscle tissue. This BCAA is found in nearly all protein sources, including brown rice, beans, nuts and whole wheat.

2. **ISOLEUCINE** This BCAA amino acid has a very similar job to leucine. Isoleucine promotes muscle recovery, regulates blood-sugar levels and stimulates HGH release. But, in terms of wound healing, isoleucine has its BCAA brothers beaten.

   Isoleucine helps in the formation of hemoglobin and is involved in the formation of blood-clots, the body's primary defense against infection through open wounds. Isoleucine is an important part of the BCAA stack. Here are the food sources you will find this BCAA in naturally: chicken, cashews, fish, almonds, eggs, lentils, liver and meat.

3. **Valine** The other BCAA that helps repair and grow muscle tissue like all 3 BCAA's, is Valine. This amino acid maintains the nitrogen balance and preserves the use of glucose, which means it will help your muscles to stay looking full. Here are the foods that offer Valine to you on a silver platter: Dairy, meat, grain, mushrooms, soy, and peanuts.

4. **Threonine** We are done with the BCAA's and onto the last essential amino acid. This amino acid mainly comes from dairy and meat, so it's tough to be a vegan and get this amino acid in your diet. This is the amino acid that binds substances together, namely collagen and elastin.

It is also essential to maintain proper protein balance. This amino acid is involved in liver functioning and lipotropic functions (when combined with aspartic acid and methionine). Threonine is also involved with the maintenance of the immune system by helping in the production of antibodies and promoting growth and activity of the thymus.

The most practical use for Threonine lies in the fact that *it allows better absorption of other nutrients*. This means protein sources containing Threonine are more bio-available than others. You can find Threonine in meat, dairy and eggs.

Non-Essential Amino Acids You Should Know About

- **Glutamine,** more commonly known as L-Glutamine, is a non-essential amino acid that is present in the body in vast quantities. Glutamine is a very important amino acid in the body. It has a lot of tasks to satisfy and without it, you would have some major health problems.

  Glutamine passes through the blood-brain barrier rather easily so it is often called brain-food. It is widely regarded as the amino acid that aids in memory and concentration. In the brain, Glutamine converts to glutamic acid, which is essential for brain function.

  It is also used in the synthesis of muscle-tissue. Yep, Glutamine is mind and body activation. It is literally one of the building blocks of the genetic code, so on a deeper note, glutamine is responsible for who and what you become. This amino acid is literally found in several strands of DNA.

  Hopefully this helps you to understand how important it is in the body. Glutamine also balances the acid/alkaline levels in your body, which means it reduces lactic acid. Lactic acid is that burning feeling near the end of a workout that takes the fire out of your muscles. So mitigating lactic acid is like Viagra for your workouts.

  Not to mention, a healthy acid/alkaline balance is crucial for good health. This amino acid even helps blunt hunger. The only issue with glutamine is that while it can do all of these amazing things, you really have no power over what your body decides to burn it for. By burn it, I mean use it as fuel.

Typically, when on a caloric surplus, your body already has so much extra glutamine that your body will even sometimes burn this amino acid before it burns carbs. The point is, there's really no reason to supplement with glutamine when your diet is in check. But that won't stop supplement companies from marketing it to you.

There is one exception to what I just said. When in a dieting phase (or a caloric deficit), your carbs are much lower than when on a bulking (caloric surplus) or maintenance phase. When you don't have as many carbs readily available, your body will automatically take fuel from different places. Your body is programed to take the most easily accessible fuels first.

In this dieting phase, if you're not careful, your body will break your muscle tissue down and burn it for fuel. The preferred fuel of must tissues is glutamine, so supplementing with glutamine during intense, elongated dieting phases will help you to hold onto your hard earned muscle while getting shredded.

I am not trying to sell you glutamine as a must have cutting supplement or telling you that it's holy; just that it could be that .01% difference that may give you the edge on retaining muscle during a cut. I know it's a catch 22; while bulking, glutamine supplementation is absolutely useless, when cutting, it does have some practical application value.

Keep in mind I'm talking about cutting sub 10% body fat, so if you're cutting from 15% to 20%, then don't worry about losing muscle until sub 10%. The supplementation of glutamine on a cut is pricey, and getting shredded is already pricey because of the food you have to eat. Buying tons of veggies and spinach gets fucking expensive after a while. Also, consider a lot of people who are getting really shredded have an online coach which can be anywhere from $150-$250 a month.

Supplementation should be the last thing on your list of crucial "Jacked & Shredded" investments. Focus on the essentials first: knowledge, diet, training, lifestyle, balance. Then you can experiment with supplements. There are large amounts of glutamine in all high protein foods, so don't stress it, just understand it.

- **Arginine,** or more commonly called L-Arginine, is an amino acid that is taken by a lot of bodybuilders as a supplement. Arginine is added as a pivotal ingredient in many supplements because of its profound nitrogen retention abilities. Nitrogen is one of the key elements in muscle protein synthesis.

  Arginine is known for enhancing the immune system and it stimulates the size and activity of the thymus gland (which is responsible for the legendary "T-cells"), which is why it's used to help aid injury recovery and to treat HIV patients.

This amino acid has hormonal release properties including the release of insulin from the pancreas, and is a huge stimulator in the manufacturing of GH from the anterior pituitary. Growth hormone is one of the most important hormones for muscle growth, so anything that stimulates GH, you want to know about and understand.

It is even linked to sexual stimulus, and it may lengthen and improve organisms, I mean orgasms. It may end up being the cure for sterility, we aren't sure yet, but it's a thing, it's a possibility. The reason it should interest you from a Jacked & Shredded standpoint is that it facilitates muscle mass gain while limiting fat storage.

Basically, it's the magical bulking supplement, because it keeps fat alive in the system and uses it. What I'm saying is that it helps convert fat into energy while allowing the food you're eating to aid your muscle growth.

Whether you're a man or woman, arginine is helpful for sexual health and performance. It increases blood flow and blood vessel health, which in turn helps you to have better blood pressure, and reduces the risk or blood clots and stroke.

I like arginine and I believe it can be beneficial in bulking or cutting. It has so many practical benefits, like the fact that it is a natural blood pressure regulator, promotor of good health, fat burner and muscle builder. If I were going to supplement an amino acid down the road, it would probably be arginine.

Again, I am still saying that supplements should be at the bottom of your priority list, but when the time comes, look into this amino acid as your friend. Make sure to do the research and get the dosage right. You can OD on arginine; it probably won't kill you but it would leave you in a world of shit, pun intended.

Always play it safe and do at least a few hours of research before going for any supplement. Here are some natural arginine sources just to tickle your fancy: whole-wheat, nuts and seeds, rice, chocolate, raisins and soy.

- **Carnitine** This little guy isn't really an amino acid but it is classified as an amino acid because of its molecular structure. It is actually known as "Vitamin BT." Carnitine comes in 4 different forms: D-carnitine, DL-carnitine, L-carnitine and Acetyl-L-carnitine (ALC). Only these last 2 forms are actually used by bodybuilders.

  Carnitine is known to aid the assistance of fat cell breakdown. It effectively helps your body to break down fat cells and burn them for energy. It seems that carnitine actually rips short-chain organic acids out of the mitochondria, which means carnitine is evicting unwelcome fat cells out of their homes and throwing them in the incinerator.

  Kids, babies, dogs, cats - Sir Carnitine does not care. He is here to burn your entire fat cell family to ashes. Carnitine may also be beneficial in preventing muscle buildup within the heart, liver and other muscles. It even improves the anti-oxidizing effect of certain vitamins, mainly vitamins C and E.

If you are looking to maintain a lean physique year-round, carnitine may be a useful supplement for you. It has been proven to show some effect on helping you to lean down and stay lean. But carnitine is found in most high protein foods, so don't go buck wild buying a bunch of carnitine to get shredded.

If you ever take up fitness as a career and your finances are directly related to your body fat levels, then I would look into carnitine as a supplement. For now, understand that this vitamin/amino acid can be found in fish, chicken, red meat and milk. Carnitine is important to understand for anyone looking to get into fitness, and build a physique.

- **Beta-Alanine** is somewhat of a popular supplement and ingredient in most pre workouts. It's what gives you that tingle and hot feeling in the body and face. Some love this feeling, I like it, and some hate it. You are about to understand it.

  Beta-Alanine is technically a non-essential beta-amino acid, but the fitness industry has hyped it up to be essential for gains. The question is, which is it really? If there was ever something that was difficult to categorize, it would be Beta-Alanine.

  It is a beta-amino acid that is somewhere between amino acid, vitamin and neurotransmitter.

"Damn scientists," right? I am not a scientist, but I am all about the current science and I believe that staying up to date on sports nutrition science is enough because being scientifically correct helps me bring results to you.

When Beta-Alanine is consumed as a dietary supplement, it passes from the bloodstream into skeletal muscle via a beta-alanine and taurine transporter that's dependent upon both sodium and chloride availability. Once it enters a muscle cell, it binds with the essential amino acid L-histidine to form dipeptide carnosine.

Fact: four weeks of six grams per day of Beta-Alanine increased the punch of amateur boxers by 20x. Since Beta-Alanine became a thing, it's been used to increase performance of muscle power output, strength, training volume, high-intensity exercise and peak oxygen uptake. Everyone from soccer players to boxers to strength athletes have seen performance gains up to 75% after 12-16 weeks of consistent use of beta-alanine.

In my opinion, this is probably one of the most track proven supplements for building muscle. So whenever the time comes to play around with supplements, look into and research Beta-Alanine. There is no doubt that this supplement increases performance and gains consistently across the board. For the whole scoop on Beta-Alanine, check out this article on bodybuilding.com

Here are some whole food sources of beta-alanine: poultry, wheat, broccoli, eggs, garlic, onion and peppers.

- **Cysteine** is your sulfur-containing friend. Our little friend here, "Cysteine" is the manufacturer of taurine, which is a component of glutathione. Glutathione protects the brain and liver from damage by way of drugs, alcohol, and other substances the body considers harmful. This amino acid's main job is to metabolize B-vitamins and detoxify the liver. You can get this amino acid from poultry, wheat, broccoli, eggs garlic, onion, and peppers.

- **HMB,** it may sound like a lifestyle clothing brand, but it's actually Beta-Hydroxy Beta-Methyl Butyrate, which is made from the essential BCAA leucine. So this little guy is an affiliate of CEO leucine. HMB plays an important role in muscle synthesis by increasing the rate of protein being used. This leads to less fat storage and contributes to the maintenance of muscle mass.

  Basically, it helps you to better absorb and take advantage of the protein you're consuming and the free amino acids in your body. This means when in a caloric deficit, HMB helps your body to preserve muscle by improving the use of free amino acids in the body. It also prevents the use of engaged amino acids (eating your own muscle) by minimizing protein breakdown.

  Now, in theory this could be a great supplement to help prevent muscle loss when cutting, right? Well, what about carnitine and glutamine? Those two offer a little more bang for your buck in terms of all of their benefits. HMB is cool, and great to understand, but I just don't believe it's a worthy investment in terms of money spent per servings vs. results.

If I were going to opt for a muscle sparing amino acid supplement, it would be either glutamine or carnitine. Personally, I don't take supplements at all, and I have been lifting for almost 11 years. If I were to look towards amino acids for supplementation, I would say carnitine would be my go to bulking supplement for its fat mobilization affects; while glutamine would be my go to cutting supplement for its muscle sparing affects and mental health.

Beta-Alanine, in my opinion, has some of the most profound effects on performance long term, as well as creatine monohydrate. By the way, this is where you can find natural sources of HMB: it's present in many foods in trace amounts with the largest amounts found in catfish, grapefruit and alfalfa.

Proclusion

Protein is something we need to survive, grow and make GAINZ. There are tons of different forms of protein, which all have their own unique abilities and amino acid breakdowns.

All protein is not made equally; it's important to know and understand this. Protein is the building block of the body, not just muscle, everything. It's important that we consume enough protein but don't go overboard on our protein intake. .8-1.2 grams of protein per pound of bodyweight is a great range to stick to.

Anything over 1.2 grams of protein per pound of bodyweight is a bit excessive, and there is absolutely no reason to ever eat twice your bodyweight in protein. Taking a look at the amino acids, it's easy to see just how powerful supplementation of isolated amino acids can be.

No, you don't necessarily need supplements, but when you have been doing this for 10+ years and have a close relationship with your physique and body chemistry, they can give you an edge.

At the end of the day, it's important to know all of this stuff, but not to take it to heart. You don't always need to be eating the highest BV protein out there. In the grand scheme of things, it won't make that big of a difference. The goal is never to be perfect but to get the right quantities of high quality protein most of the time.

I am a big fan of L-Arginine and Beta-Alanine, they work well for me, always have. To be honest though, I don't recommend any pre workout supplementation of any kind unless you work a manual labor job. Those who work manual labor jobs may benefit from a pre workout containing these amino acids along with being caffeine ambidextrous. Otherwise these workers may not have the energy to lift afterwards.

I can tell you this from experience. I have worked construction in the heat, and you don't have anything left for a workout afterwards. During the time I worked construction, pre workout was much more helpful than at any other point in my life. Learn, but don't marry; data and information changes every day. We conduct new research and discover new things about protein and the body on a monthly basis. It's important to keep up with current data, which is why I have made that easy for you.

FAT

Fat is the overlooked macronutrient that people often crucify by saying fat makes you fat. Fat does not make you fat, eating too much food makes you fat, whether it's protein, fat, carbs or a mix of just too many calories in general.

Fat is a more flexible macronutrient than protein, but you do need to make sure, in any case, that you're getting enough fat in your diet. Your fat intake should be anywhere from 20% to 35% of your total calories for the day. I recommend aiming towards the middle of that set point around 25-30% of your total daily calories.

I would never recommend you ever to drop lower than .25 grams of fat per pound of bodyweight, and there really isn't any reason to ever venture above .75 grams of fat per pound of bodyweight. Again, just as protein, your fat needs to be based off of your bodyweight, age, gender, body type, and goals. Here is a list of things that depend on fat:

- Growth and development.

- Energy production (fat is the most concentrated source of energy).

- Absorbing certain vitamins (like vitamins A, D, E, K and even carotenoids).

- Providing essential cushioning for the organs.

- Maintenance of the cell membranes.

- Fat is the macronutrient that provides taste, consistency, and stability to foods.

Here is a list of foods fat that are high in fat: meat, poultry, nuts, milk products, butters and margarines, oils, lard, fish, grain products and salad dressings. We have three main types of fat, saturated fat, unsaturated fat, and trans fat.

Saturated fat (found in foods like meat, butter, lard, and cream) and trans fat (found in baked goods, snack foods, fried foods, and margarines) have been shown to increase your risk for heart disease. Replacing saturated and trans fat in your diet with unsaturated fat (found in foods like olive oil, avocados, nuts, and canola oil), has been shown decrease the risk of developing heart disease.

Contrary to popular belief, some saturated fat in the diet is heathy. You are going to have saturated fats in your meats, eggs, poultry and fish. Not a lot, but you will run into some, and this amount is good. You want to try to stay away from overly fatty beef and steak and fatback.

Saturated fat in higher quantities is not really something you want to consume often. Saturated fat can't all be bad because the type of saturated fat you get from coconut oil is literally considered to be one of the healthiest fats in the world. So saturated fat isn't bad; you just don't want to base your diet off of it.

Monounsaturated Fat

This is one of the two unsaturated fats that you want to consume. This type of fat is found in avocados, nuts, and vegetable oils such as canola, olive and peanut. By eating foods that are high in monounsaturated fats, you will be helping yourself lower, and keep in check, your LDL cholesterol.

You will also be helping to keep your HDL cholesterol levels higher. Paying attention to this sort of stuff is going to help you perform better, have more natural energy, be more clearly minded, and live much longer.

Polyunsaturated fat

You will find this type of fat in vegetable oils like safflower, sunflower, sesame, soybean, and corn oils. This is also the main fat found in seafood. Eating polyunsaturated fat will also help you to lower LDL cholesterol levels. There are two types of fat found in polyunsaturated fat.

- **Omega-3 fatty acids** are fatty acids found in plant foods such as soybean oil, canola oil, walnuts and flaxseed. You can also find these fatty acids in fatty fish and shellfish as eicosapentaenoic acid (EPA) and docosahexaenoic acid (DHA). Salmon, anchovies herring, sardines, Pacific oysters, trout, Atlantic mackerel and Pacific mackerel are all high in EPA and DHA and lower in mercury.

- **Omega-6 fatty acids** Omega-6 fatty acids you need - they are essential fatty acids. Omega-6 fatty acids are necessary for human health, but the body can't produce these fatty acids. Just as omega-3 fatty acids, omega-6 fatty acids play a crucial role in brain function, and normal growth and development. Omega-6 fatty acids are a type of polyunsaturated fatty acid (PUFA) and they help stimulate skin and hair growth, maintain bone health, regulate metabolism, and maintain the reproductive system.

What the Crap is Trans-fat

Trans-fat is your worst nightmare. Trans-fat is a screwed up trans-unsaturated fatty acid with a double bond between two carbon atoms. This fat molecule tends to stick along the lining of cells, where it is then attacked by free radicals that damage the rest of the cell. Eating trans-fat is basically like inviting a criminal into your house who wants to steal your gains, your health, and your life because he can.

The process of creating manmade trans-fat is a process called hydrogenation. This is done by adding hydrogen to liquid fat sources to make them more solid. Trans-fat is widely associated with coronary heart disease and is a leading cause of death in Western nations. Trans-fats are edible, but do you want cancer on purpose?

This stuff lowers your good HDL cholesterol and brings up the bad LDL cholesterol. On the 16th of June, 2015, the FDA finally put their foot down saying chemically altered trans-fats were not safe to consume and set a 3-year time limit for their removal from all processed foods. Companies with a good heart, who care about the world, stopped using trans-fats. On the contrary, a ton of other companies gave no shits and are riding the money train straight through until June 16, 2018.

Oddly enough, countries other than the "MERCA"

have already enforced limits on trans-fat content. We discovered trans-fat in 1910 and we found we could use it to make much more profit; just hydrogenate the soybean oil and now we have 2 uses for soybeans - protein and fatty oil.

Try to minimize your eating of anything that says "partially hydrogenated oils" on the label. You will be unpleasantly surprised with how many things actually have trans-fats in them. Looking for products with no trans-fat on the label is definitely a good idea. You can't make gains if you're dead.

Trans-fats have no place in the body of a physique builder, or anyone else. They will decrease your performance and make you feel like poop. It's easy to see why there is so much bad health in the world with the combination of HFCS and trans-fats are being consumed more than complex carbs and healthy fatty acids.

Be aware: foods can be listed as "trans-fat free" if they contain less than .5 grams per serving. Trans-fats can be found in many foods such as fried foods like doughnuts, and baked goods including cakes, pie crusts, biscuits, frozen pizza, cookies, crackers, stick margarines and other spreads. That's not all, just an example.

Oddly enough, an unmolested version of trans-fat is found in nature. Dairy fat and grass fed meats contain a pretty high amount of trans-fatty acids. The thing is, naturally occurring trans-fat is good for you, it's the manmade, hydrogen infused trans-fats that kill us. Animal fats are actually very healthy for us, so don't listen to what anyone else says.

Medium-chain Triglycerides are more commonly known as the "the good saturated fat." These fats seem to do very miraculous things in both the health world and the fitness world. MCT's are found naturally in milk fat, palm oil, and coconut oil.

One really cool thing to note is that MCT's help to prevent diabetes from ever becoming forever chained to you because they increase your body's tolerance to carbohydrates. This is because using MCT's as an alternative source of fuel tends to drop your blood sugar levels just enough to give your pancreas a break from producing insulin.

This is why I preach a balanced diet so often. Without good fats like these, you may end up with some issues, the same issues that most Americans are dealing with, like diabetes. MCT's are rapidly absorbed and oxidized. They are absorbed into the bloodstream as MCFAs (Medium Chain Fatty Acids) and metabolized as quickly as glycogen.

It is possible that MCFA's may enhance performance by sparing glycogen utilized during weight training. I am not saying this is a fact, but I do believe it to be true. I have seen many bodybuilders who chose to diet using the Keto approach, which basically means a diet where your body switches its energy source from glucose from carbs, to ketones from fat.

This is another reason that trying to lower your blood glucose levels as a means to burn fat by replacing carbs with fat doesn't work. While it is good to have these fats in your diet, your body will always find a way to use the calories you're eating. This is why I preach about thermodynamics and calories; you can't trick your body into burning more fat by switching one macronutrient for another, but I digress. MCT's could possibly save the world, and realistically improve our gains. It's one of my favorite molecules out of any macronutrient.

MCT's may cure Alzheimer's?

As crazy as this sounds, I remember when I was 14 years old and I was studying the effects MCT's may have on the cognitive functions of the brain. My grandma was starting to show signs of different pathetical illnesses, ever so slightly. I knew at 14 that being into fitness was my way of helping people, hopefully one day millions, but at the moment just my grandma.

Scientists have been looking into this for a long time now. In animals, MCT supplementation can improve brain function, reduce Alzheimer's-like pathology, and enhance learning in animals. Here is a link to many studies on the effects of triglycerides on age-related cognitive decline in older subjects.

This is my take on the studies, and my theory: Over time, eating a diet high in refined sugars like HFCS, low in protein, and low in amounts of high quality fat, diminishes the brain's ability to make use of glucose. Now, I believe this happens naturally overtime. However, I believe that the amount of time your brain stays healthy is predicated on a balanced diet, to put this simply.

MCT's may slow the onset of diseases like Alzheimer's, but we aren't completely sure just yet. The thing is, the brain's main source of fuel is glucose. In patients with mild cognitive impairment or dementia, brain cells lose some of their ability to use glucose as a fuel. This effect may accelerate disease progression, worsen cognitive abilities and increase Alzheimer's disease pathology, all stuff we don't want our grandmas and grandpas to have.

MCT's may be the substitute to glucose. Once digested, they are broken down by the liver into ketone bodies, which are then released into the bloodstream to provide an alternative source of fuel for the body and brain. Ketones are pretty cool. Here are more studies in case I have intrigued you.

A Positron Emission Tomography (PET) Study Evaluating Brain Metabolism of a Medical Food in Alzheimer's Disease (AD)

Retrospective Cohort Study Of The Efficacy Of Axona® (Medium Chain Triglycerides) In Patients With Alzheimer's Disease (ACT)

Study to Evaluate Coconut Oil for Alzheimer's Disease

Caprylic Triglyceride for Treatment of Cognitive Impairments in Multiple Sclerosis

Effect of a Medium Chain Triglyceride Supplemented Diet on Cognitive Function and Brain Activation in Type 1 Diabetes.

MCT's for Bodybuilding and Performance

MCT's bypass the digestion process that longer chain fatty acids go through. This means MCT's provide quick energy and are less likely to be stored in the fat cells as a result. When MCT's are metabolized, they behave more like a carbohydrate than a fat. We know that the fuel of preference for the body is carbohydrates.

MCT's are not like other fats because MCT oil does not go through the lymphatic system. These guys are transported directly to the liver where they are metabolized, so they release energy like a carbohydrate and create lots of ketones which can be used as fuel in the process.

Our bodies are 70% water, and fat is not very soluble in water; your body has to go through this super crazy digestive process to absorb and metabolize fat. Your gall bladder produces bile to help dissolve the long chain triglycerides, generating these tiny little fat droplets called micelles. Then it's your intestines' job to transport these fats to your lymphatic system. Then fat is finally passed into the bloodstream through the thoracic duct, where they are either burned or stored as body fat.

Your body has a very frustrating task metabolizing these fats so sometimes, when on a caloric surplus, they are more easily stored as body fat than protein and carbs. These fats are found in everything from animal fat to dairy products. I am not telling you they're bad, just that you should be sparing with them.

Aim to get more of your calories from MCT's and carbs. MCT's are not so hard to deal with, not like LCTs. MCT's can be used to fuel the muscle by the use of ketones. Some MCT's are used for thermogenesis, and a portion is converted to ATP, the energy currency of the cell - all stuff you want to happen. These types of fats are less likely to add to your fat cells and more likely to keep you from gaining them. MCT's are good fats, so eat them!

9 Fatty Acids that are Worth Talking About

1. **Alpha Linoleic Acid** is one of two essential fatty acids (EFA's). We call them essential fatty acids because they are essential for our health. These fatty acids must be acquired through diet; your body doesn't make much of them.

   ALA is part of the happy omega-3 fatty acid family next door. You can find this fatty acid in seeds such as chia and flaxseed; you can also find ALA in walnuts and many common vegetable oils. This doesn't make me anymore of a fan of vegetable oil, I would get this fat from seeds and nuts.

I don't like vegetable oils because most of the time they have been molested and chemically changed. Not saying vegetable oils are bad, just that it's difficult to find unmolested vegetable oils that aren't hydrogenated to shit. ALA has been shown to help decrease the risk of heart attack and heart disease.

Basically it helps to keep you heart healthy, which is a characteristic of an omega-3 fatty acid if there ever was one. ALA greatly reduces high blood pressure. It may even help improve lung function in some people with asthma. I have asthma, so this is especially appealing to me. It's great for your cardiovascular system as well, and may lower bad LDL cholesterol while raising the good LDL. Here are some great natural sources of ALA.

- *Flaxseeds, and flaxseed oil*
- *Canola (rapeseed) oil*
- *Soybeans and soybean oil*
- *Pumpkin seeds and pumpkin seed oil*
- *Perilla seed oil*
- *Tofu*
- *Walnuts and walnut oil*

Here are all the studies that support the claims I just made for all of you anal science guys, P.S. I'm just like you, I need to know that info is accurate, so here you go:

Marangoni F, Colombo C, Martiello A, Poli A, Paoletti R,

Galli C. Levels of the n-3 fatty acid eicosapentaenoic acid in addition to those of alpha linolenic acid are significantly raised in blood lipids by the intake of four walnuts a day in humans. *Nutr Metab Cardiovasc Dis.*2007;17(6):457-461.

Okamoto M, Misunobu F, Ashida K, Mifune T, Hosaki Y, Tsugeno H, et al. Effects of dietary supplementation with n-3 fatty acids compared with n-6 fatty acids on bronchial asthma. *Int Med.* 2000;39(2):107-111.

Pan A, Chen M, Chowdhury R, et al. a-Linolenic acid and risk of cardiovascular disease: a systematic review and meta-analysis. *Am J Clin Nutr.* 2012; 96(6):1262-1273.

Djousse L, Arnett DK, Carr JJ, et al. Dietary linolenic acid is inversely associated with calcified atherosclerotic plaque in the coronary arteries: the National Heart, Lung, and Blood Institute Family Heart Study. *Circulation.* 2005;111:2921-2926.

Since there are so many studies, I am going to link you to the page that sites all of them. UMM.EDU

ALA for Bodybuilding

When ALA is present in high quantities it acts as an antioxidant, even though it is an omega-3 fatty acid. Alpha-Lipoic Acid has the ability to deactivate both fat and water soluble free radicals (like the build-up of excess minerals underneath the surface of your skin), which means it can protect both lipoproteins and membranes. No other anti-oxidant can do this.

What I am saying is ALA is a toxin fighter, it takes your toxins and breaks their noses, then bitch slaps them, then curb stomps them. That's pretty much what ALA does to free radicals. Just so you understand what a free radical is, it represents the aging of your cells, the oxidation of your cells, and the destruction of your cells.

So when I talk about free radicals, those are the things that kill you, your muscles and your brain, and not necessarily in that order. The more we learn about stopping free radicals, the longer we stay healthy in mind and body.

In essence, when you eat things that create free radicals in your body, you are speeding up the process of the aging and determination of your cells.

Eating things like trans-fats and isolated fructose has this effect on the body. ALA is a fighter of the free radical just like every other antioxidant. When you think antioxidant, think anti-oxidation of your cells, anti-aging, and the defense of your cellular life. ALA is on the forefront of this cellular defense.

When people are eating things that cause free radicals to form, and disregarding the foods that provide antioxidants to fight the free radicals, it's no wonder we are obese, diseased and unhappy; we are doing it to ourselves, we just can't see the destruction up close.

ALA is something you need to know about. Similar to MCT's, ALA has been shown to actually reverse the damage in aging cells of the brain. This study was published in the journal *Proceedings of the National Academy of Science* in February of 2015.

For the same reasons, some people use it to improve performance in memory tasks by lowering oxidative damage and improving mitochondrial function. Here are the practical reasons that may intrigue you. This is a great supplement to take if you are someone that believes in vitamin, mineral and antioxidant supplementation.

- Improves physique

- Combats free radicals +++
- Protects our genetic material
- Slows aging
- Protects against heart disease
- Protects against cancer
- Improves skin and helps erase wrinkles
- Regulates blood sugar in diabetics
- Protects the liver
- May be used as a treatment for stroke

Hopefully you are starting to understand how powerful it can be to have the knowledge to build a healthy eating lifestyle that will benefit you for the rest of your life. ALA has to be my favorite fatty acid supplement because of its crazy ability to do so many positive things for the body.

This is definitely something you should consider: it even plays a role in healthy levels of testosterone. I am sure I have your attention now. ALA supplementation is something that I strongly recommend if you ever worry about any of the things I mentioned about it. You can't go wrong with ALA.

2. **EPA** or Eicosapentaenoic acid, is another fatty acid that's part of the omega-3 fatty acid group. EPA is a polyunsaturated fatty acid that you can get from eating oily fish or fish oil. Here are some great food sources of EPA: cod, liver, hearing, mackerel, salmon, menhaden and sardine.

    All of the omega-3 fatty acids exhibit similar miraculous results. This makes sense because they're all chemically very similar, like three brothers. The human body actually converts ALA to EPA. So whether you eat EPA or not, your body is going to make you some damn EPA in its synthesizing lab.

Here's the thing, remember a couple of minutes ago when you were learning about the amazing effects of ALA? Well, if you're not getting enough EPA, your body is going to convert some of the ALA you have just consumed into EPA.

Now, there is no need to worry because all three omega-3 fatty acids are awesome, but it would be more beneficial to give your body what it wants and needs instead of forcing it to synthesize it. Here's the funny part: the 3rd omega-3 fatty acid we will be talking about is a precursor of EPA and it's called DHA (Docosahexaenoic Acid).

So, if you don't get all three omega-3 fatty acids, your body is going to pull EPA from ALA, and DHA from EPA. It's a very metabolically expensive performance for your body to do so, and while it does work, it's not super-efficient. This is why omega-3 acid supplements are helpful.

Now that we have discussed the links between the three brothers, let's talk about all the benefits of EPA. How is it that we are always asking about benefits from the companies we work for, but never from the foods we habitually eat? Ever thought about that? You will never see those job benefits if you're dead, and if you're living off of pills for heart, blood pressure, stress, depression, anxiety, diabetes, liver disease, etc., are you really alive?

EPA has something to say about all of that. You

know how children need omega-3 fatty acids to ensure proper development of their brains? How many of us actually ate any fish, or took omega-3 as a child? I can't say I did, not until I was about 12, and I do have some attention disorders. EPA has been shown to possibly reduce ADHD symptoms. I can tell you from personal experience, that when my diet is bad, i.e. when I eat simple sugars all day and not enough healthy fats like EPA and ALA, I can tell a notable difference in my productivity. I tend to space out much, much more and want to take naps, and I am not very creative. I just feel like being a lazy potato. Being a lazy potato tends to breed more lazy potato behavior.

Luckily paying attention to this is what I do, so I will never let this go on longer than half a day. Want to feel better, have more energy, be more mentally sharp, and less foggy? Eat less refined carbs and more omega-3 fats.

Some other studies showed that EPA reduces the symptoms of depression. I can attribute to this as well: at 13, my health and mood took a turn for the worst. My daily life consisted of skittles, game fuel Mountain Dew, and Hot Cheetos. I became wildly overweight and deficient of muscle mass. My metabolism was dropping, my hormones were whack, and my sugar levels were all over the place. I very nearly committed suicide, and then I decided to change.

Naturally this meant a more balanced diet which included healthy fats. By 15, my depression had completely subsided and I attribute a portion of this to my reduction in processed carb sources and my uptake of healthy fats such as EPA and ALA. Why am I telling you this? Because it could save your life as well.

It could also get you the body and mindset you want. One more obvious benefit of fish oil is its stand against heart disease. Yes, just as ALA counters heart disease, EPA also fights the same fight. Eat your trout, albacore tuna and salmon! Rheumatoid Arthritis may even be taken out by EPA. It has been tested time and time again, and seems to reduce the inflammation that RA causes in the joints. It also may combat Lupus by reducing fatigue and joint pain.

It has so many other great qualities, but these are all the main things that would be of help to you. Some of these disorders can greatly affect your gym performance, work performance and mindset every day. EPA plays a big role in autoimmune disease relief as well as brain fuel.

In terms of making muscle gains, EPA works within the cell membrane to enhance insulin's ability to transport nutrients. This process of EPA and DHA doing their brain fueling and muscle nutrient fueling, decreases in athletes over 30. So for those of you that are 30 and older, I strongly recommend omega-3 fatty acids for several reasons.

Arguably, omega-3 fatty acids are most important for young children and adults over the age of 30 but consider this - if you are between the ages of 16 and 28, you're in your prime stages of muscle growth. So if you want to maximize gains, omega-3 is your friend.

EPA is the only nutrient found to de-activate the major molecular pathway of muscle breakdown (catabolism). In conditions such as cancer, HIV and severe infection, your muscle wasting pathways are open for business, which means you're catabolic. When on a caloric deficit, your body opens the same muscle wasting pathways to burn your hard earned muscle for fuel.

So when you're cutting, looking to get shredded, EPA may be very helpful in stopping you from losing muscle. I believe EPA and glutamine are very helpful together when on a cut and looking to retain as much muscle as possible. I know I have been talking a lot about supplementation these past couple of pages, so please understand that I am not telling you that you need all of these nutrients in supplement form.

I am telling you what they could be used for once your diet is in check. I would use EPA as a supplement year around, but it would be especially helpful to take advantage of during around the final 8-10 weeks leading up to a bodybuilding show or a fitness photoshoot when you're on a caloric deficit and sub 10% body fat.

Omega-3 supplementation would be a better idea for year-round health for the mind and muscles. At the end of the day, EPA can do some pretty cool stuff, and it definitely should have a part in every healthy diet. If you want studies, here are my sources.

Bodybuilding

Health

3. **DHA** or Docosahexaenoic acid is the third omega-3 fatty acid out of the bunch. It is a primary structural component of the human brain, cerebral cortex, skin, sperm, testicles and retina. Your body can synthesize it from ALA or you can obtain it from food.

    You can get it from a fish oil supplement or algae oil. DHA is critical for optimal brain health and function at all ages of life. We now have proof that DHA can not only provide brain boosting benefits for aging adults, but also for young adults, even down to infants. DHA is critical for neurological and visual development in infants, and we have never thought of it as an ingredient in baby food, until now.

    Maybe the fact that some people grow up to need glasses at a young age is predicated on nutritional deficiencies as an infant? I am not a doctor or a scientist, so please don't take anything I say as the absolute gospel, I could be wrong. My theory is that we will have more healthy babies both cognitively and regarding vision once we reestablish what baby formula should be.

    There is a reason why mother's breast milk is perfect for a baby. It has all the essential fatty acids a baby needs along with the right amounts of carbs, the right amino acid breakdown, and casein plus whey protein. We are still trying to figure out how to replicate or one-up this natural baby food today. Enough about babies.

DHA is a strong contender against depression, post-traumatic stress disorder, and possibly Alzheimer's disease. It's well known by doctors that omega-3 fatty acids improve brain function, decrease inflammation, reduce the possibility of fatal heart attack and stroke, improve the outcome of autoimmune diseases, and improve vision. DHA also has a lot to do with the CNS. It is a big factor in the brain sending signals to the muscles.

DHA is found mainly in the motor control areas of the brain, which play a huge role in muscle development, including memory, social development and behavior. No wonder we are all weird, immobile, uncoordinated, and skinny, now it all makes sense! Most of us have been super deficient in essential omega-3 fatty acids for years.

It turns out that a lot of kids with attention disorders just didn't get enough DHA and omega-3's in their diets early on. That may be the same issue with socially awkward kids. If you are super skinny, or chubby with no muscle, socially awkward, and have an attention disorder, listen carefully to what I am about to say. You will probably be written off as partially slow, hyperactive, a socially awkward case, etc. You will probably be then offered Ritalin and Zoloft.

This makes me very fucking mad, you are not some weird kid that needs drugs to be normal. Drugs never solve anything, they don't. Both of these compounds affect the chemicals in the brain. Great, now you're on drugs like the rest of the world. Maybe instead of drugs, try dropping your simple sugar uptake, and adding in omega-3 fatty acid packed foods, omega-3 fatty acid supplements are a great idea.

I am not big on pumped up, highly marketed bodybuilding supplements, but omega-3 fatty acids are something that are essential that most of us need much more of. Do you know that Ritalin is a stimulant just like cocaine? Of course it's going to change your brain chemistry, stimulants can change everyone's brain chemistry, but are they fixing things? Nope. Do you know that Zoloft is something that helps you relax and be happy, but that weed does this much better?

So if this is what we are trying to do, why don't we just put the weird kids on cocaine so they become the cool kids, and teach the depressed kids to smoke weed so they will be medicated and happy? Oops, we already do this, don't we? My bad.

I think we are all missing the point here. We are trying to medicate what is not broken. We are not fixing problems, we are just covering them with smoke and mirrors. I was a depressed, socially awkward kid at 13, but I had reasons to be. I had been put on Zoloft and Ritalin. Zoloft made me want to kill myself, and Ritalin turned me into a lifeless zombie who was better than anyone in his class at math, in other words, I was on crack.

Maybe I just needed more omega-3 fatty acids and some protein in my diet. Parents that are letting their kids eat shit all day are doing them a disservice. Tell them they can eat *this* way and become *this* type of person, and eat better and become another type of person because it's a fact.

You are what you eat, literally. Is this making sense? I would never have been able to focus for one second to write this book had I not changed my eating habits and physical activity at age 13. I do not take any medications today, and I am more mentally sharp than ever. To think my second grade teacher told my parents that I was slow. I am not slow; my brain requires more fatty acids then some people.

DHA for Bodybuilding

This stuff is great for your joints, especially if you do isolation work in the gym, i.e. skull crushers, close grip bench, dips, behind the head shoulder press, leg curls or leg extensions.

These movements are all very tough on your joints and after years of doing them, you will most likely have massive joint pain and discomfort. And you will probably blame it on the conventional bench press, squat and deadlift, just so you can then go on and do more of what beats up your joints and ligaments. Omega-3's have shown time and time again to reduce inflammation in the joints in only a matter of weeks.

So do two things for me if you are having joint pains in the gym: chill out with these accessory movements and start supplementing with omega-3 fatty acids. Oh, and do your research on the brands and quality of the product, that does make a difference. This is a supplement I suggest for anybody, year-round. It is even more helpful when cutting on a caloric deficit.

On a caloric deficit, your joints have less calories and eventually less fat to cushion the beating you throw them at the gym. Protecting yourself from injury with omega-3 fatty acids is a fabulous idea. DHA is also a natural testosterone booster for men, and as an estrogen blocker, it does exactly the opposite for women. Basically, it's just good for your hormones. Without adequate amounts of DHA and EPA, your body is not going to be efficient in its testosterone production.

So DHA basically has three great muscle building advantages: it increases the strength of the pathway between mind and muscle, helps prevent injury at the gym, and helps to elevate testosterone. This stuff is awesome. Omega-3 fatty acids should not be overlooked in bodybuilding or in a healthy lifestyle.

4. **Linoleic Acid (LA)** is a polyunsaturated omega-6 fatty acid, not to be confused with Alpha Linoleic Acid. LA is an essential fatty acid we must get from food. You can find this omega-6 fatty acid in many vegetable oils, especially safflower and sunflower oils.

    It occurs naturally in the body, but if you aren't getting enough of it, you will be dealing with things like dry hair, hair loss and poor wound healing. LA is something used in beauty products and soups. It is also used as an anti-inflammatory and in acne reduction.

    Basically, if you have dry skin, wrinkles or acne, look towards LA for help. This is your skin care fatty acid. I know from personal experience that working out and sweating a lot tends to give you acne both on your face, and annoyingly, on your chest, shoulders and upper back. Besides that, we all want to look as young and healthy as possible.

Brushing up on your LA at a young age may help your skin and hair stay healthier longer. Please do your research on the amount of LA you should take for your age and bodyweight, gender etc. This stuff can be toxic in high levels. At the end of the day, we all want great skin whether we are 16 or 61, and some of us don't have perfect skin genetics.

5. **GLA** or Gamma Linolenic Acid is an omega-6 fatty acid with some intriguing history. It's most commonly found in seeds of the evening primrose plant. Native Americans used it to reduce swelling. They were actually brilliant with their medical administrations, given their time period.

    There is a reason it took on the name "king's cure all". It's also pretty easy to get your hands on some; you can get it from most vegetable oils, and evening primrose oil, borage seed oil and blackcurrant seed oil capsules, all found at most health foods stores and online. This omega-6 FA is essential for brain function, skin growth, hair growth, skeletal reproductive health, and even regulating your metabolism.

    Pretty important stuff. Just like the omega-3 fatty acid group, this omega-6 has the ability to help combat arthritis and diabetic neuropathy. My advice is just to eat more vegetables. Most people aren't deficient in GLA, but it can be helpful to understand and know its part in a healthy diet. GLA also helps against allergies, I hate allergies. GLA, like LA, helps keep your skin in great condition and aids in blood pressure regulation. What are the odds?

Hopefully you know by now that essential fatty acids will keep your blood pressure in check. The main benefit of GLA that has my attention, is its ability to improve stress reactivity and performance, attenuated blood pressure and heart rate to stress, increased skin temperature, and improved task performance.

Do you know how important stress management is? I could practically write an entire book on stress management. Stress is a necessary part of life, but those who consume only sugar and are deficient in EFA's like GLA, may have a much harder time not attacking innocent people when shit hits the fan. The more stress you can handle, the more pressure you can deal with while staying calm and collective, and the more productive you will be in life.

Productivity is a big indicator of success in whatever you're doing. If you're not productive and not great under stress, you're fucked in today's world. Do you see now why being healthy and capitalizing on your nutrition is crucial to your performance and success in life? You should! GLA has been widely regarded as one of the most powerful omega-6 fatty acids for a while now. So if you need its super powers, don't hesitate to get the hookup from your friendly doctor.

Which reminds me, please talk to your doctor

before you start supplementing with anything powerful like GLA or LA. Here are some studies to tickle your fancy:

Cameron, M., & Gagnier, J. (2011, February 16). Herbal therapy for rheumatoid arthritis. Phytotherapy Research, 23, 1647-1662. Retrieved from http://deepblue.lib.umich.edu/bitstream/handle/2027.42/64567/3006_ftp.pdf?sequence=1

Ehrlich, S. (2011). Gamma linolenic acid. Retrieved fromhttp://umm.edu/health/medical/altmed/supplement/gammalinolenic-acid

Kapoor, R., & Huang, R. S. (2006, December). Gamma linolenic acid: an anti-inflammatory omega-6 fatty acid. Current Pharmaceutical Biotechnology, 7(6), 531-534. Retrieved from http://www.ncbi.nlm.nih.gov/pubmed/17168669.

6. **DGLA** or Dihomo-γ-linolenic acid is an omega-6 fatty acid that nobody can pronounce. You can find this unpronounceable EFA in plant-based oils. This O6FA does all of the same cool stuff that the other omega-6 fatty acids do so well, like reduce inflammation, keep your skin heathy, keep the brain healthy, etc.

   The thing that I want you to know about DGLA is that it likes to kill tumor cells. It has strong anti-tumor effects and kicks the shit out of any tumor that wants to make a home in your body. It has the ability to inhibit both motility and invasiveness of human colon cancer cells by increasing the expression of something called E-cadherin, which keeps things from going bad in your cells.

   When free radicals and lipid peroxidation are generated by PUFA's, these guys have the ability to suck the life out of tumors, leaving them empty of energy, which brings about the death of the tumor. DGLA is the big proponent of this fight against tumors.

Here is the thing: I know we aren't all sitting here thinking about tumor growth because it sucks to think about that. The fact is, it happens, sometimes to you, sometimes to your kids or parents. Health needs to come before gains. If you have a tumor, you won't be making as many gains in the gym because you will be dealing with the tumor.

Understanding omega-6 fatty acids and their importance may prevent you from ever getting a tumor or help you move onto the natural path of destroying this evil with a little more confidence than before. With the knowledge of these fatty acids, we have the power to ward off cancer, eradicate tumors, stay younger longer, build more muscle, have a more productive and successful life, keep ourselves from getting injured, and so much more.

Guys, this is the stuff that could save millions of people. It's up to us to get the true information out there. We who are obsessed with having low body fat and big muscles, performing super human lifts, taking our health to another level - it's our responsibility to make an impact.

I'm not just writing a book, I am writing a guide, a how to book on how to become an elite human. How to drop all of the bullshit and practice the truth. DGLA, and the rest of the EFA's are much more important to you than you may have noted before reading this book. Links to multiple studies.

7. **Arachidonic Acid** (AA) is another polyunsaturated omega-6 fatty acid. AA is abundant in the brain, muscles and liver. Yes, this omega-6 has a lot to do with muscles. Skeletal muscles are an especially active site of AA, with around 10-20% of the fatty acid content on average.

What I am about to talk about will seem like a big juicy retraction because I have talking about joint inflammation, and how fatty acids can reduce it. Well, not all inflammation is bad. What am I talking about, you ponder? I am talking about post-workout muscle inflammation.

Post-workout inflammation is very important regarding hypertrophy (the building of muscle). I am sure you are familiar with the post-workout feels. The sore muscles, the hot muscles, the depleted feeling, etc. It seems pretty simple; you work out hard, you get sore, and you build bigger, stronger muscles! Well, unfortunately it's not that simple my friend. You have things like growth hormone, and IFG-1 hormones that come into play when thinking about muscle building.

There are certain neurological pathways that need to be initiated within your muscle to bind these exercise-responsive hormones like GH and IFG-1. Here is the interesting part: your body's process of binding hormones in order to synthesize amino acids to build muscle, doesn't just happen on its own. Your nervous system has some involvement here, there is some neurotransmission action going on. AA is like a messenger; it makes sure that the transmissions come across.

Once the signals are sent to where they need to be,

the body then starts the elaborate and delicate process of protein synthesis. This is where your nitrogen from amino acids is linearly arranged into structural proteins through the involvement of RNA and other various enzymes. The thing is, protein synthesis is muscle growth.

The more efficient you can make the process of getting protein to protein synthesis, the better your body will be at building muscle. Basically, it helps you get to the muscle building state; it strengthens the signaling from a to b that needs to happen in order to get to protein synthesis.

This is definitely a supplement to look into if you are not getting enough omega-6 fatty acids in your diet. What you should do is simply eat more foods containing omega-6 fatty acids, and eat more foods containing AA.

This stuff is part of a ton of fat sources, so chances are you are already getting it. But just in case you're wondering, here is a list of foods where you can get your AA.

Red Meat – Especially fatty red meat
White Meat – Chicken, duck & wild fowl
Dairy – Any animal milk
Eggs
Cheeses – Especially hard cheeses
Certain fish – Tilapia, catfish, yellowtail

The issue with AA is that it's double sided; if you don't work out hard then you don't need it, and you don't even want it. This is why it's impossible to say one thing is either healthy or unhealthy. To just simply say AA is healthy or unhealthy is incorrect.

AA can only be categorized as healthy or unhealthy based on a person by person basis. It would be difficult to completely avoid AA altogether, but if you aren't breaking down your muscles constantly or getting injured a lot, you probably don't need it.

Chronic inflammation happens a lot in people with heart disease, in many cancers and Alzheimer's disease. Inflammation is categorized as redness, heat, swelling and pain. If you have any of these diseases, or any neuropathic or chronic inflammation, stay away from AA and food sources that contain it.

If you have any of those diseases, you need to opt for the fatty acids that reduce inflammation in the body. While AA helps with the process in rebuilding the muscle, if you are not someone who works the muscles hard several days a week, I would consider AA to be extremely unhealthy for you in many ways.

On the contrary, AA is great for anyone building muscle, i.e. bodybuilders and powerlifters. Isn't it interesting that what is healthy for a high performance athlete could equally hurt a normal sedentary person? This is why I get so mad about someone going on TV and blankly stating *oh, eggs are bad for you, cheese is bad for you, red meats are bad for you*. Nope, these things are bad for you if you're lazy.

You would be surprised at how many foods are "bad for you" when you're sedentary. The thing is, someone who is aerobically and muscularly conditioned, someone who gets a good amount of physical activity and lifts weight has a completely different body chemistry than someone who doesn't do those things.

The even better part is that the physical, weight-lifting person will outperform the non-physical person in every aspect of life – work performance, focus, mental clarity, heart health, sex drive, confidence, happiness, longevity, etc. Someone who pays attention to their body chemistry and stays active is tapping into their true potential as a human, while the sedentary person is wasting their potential.

So, if you are a healthy lifter looking to build more muscle with no inflammatory or neuropathic diseases, eat more foods with AA and make some more gains. Studies are listed below.

Andersson, A., A. Sjodin, A. Hedman, R. Olsson, and B. Vessby. Fatty acid profile of skeletal muscle phospholipids in trained and untrained young men. Am J Physiol Endocrinol Metab. 279:E744-751, 2000.

Aronson, D., M. D. Boppart, S. D. Dufresne, R. A. Fielding, and L. J. Goodyear. Exercise stimulates c-Jun NH2 kinase activity and c-Jun transcriptional activity in human skeletal muscle. Biochem Biophys Res Commun. 251:106-110, 1998.

Boppart, M. D., D. Aronson, L. Gibson, R. Roubenoff, L. W. Abad, J. Bean, L. J. Goodyear, and R. A. Fielding. Eccentric exercise markedly increases c-Jun NH(2)-terminal kinase activity in human skeletal muscle. J Appl Physiol. 87:1668-1673, 1999.

Boppart, M. D., S. Asp, J. F. Wojtaszewski, R. A. Fielding, T. Mohr, and L. J. Goodyear. Marathon running transiently increases c-Jun NH2-terminal kinase and p38 activities in human skeletal muscle. J Physiol. 526 Pt 3:663-669, 2000.

Glass, D. J. Molecular mechanisms modulating muscle mass. Trends Mol Med. 9:344-350, 2003.

Griendling, K. K., D. Sorescu, B. Lassegue, and M. Ushio-Fukai. Modulation of protein kinase activity and gene expression by reactive oxygen species and their role in vascular physiology and pathophysiology. Arterioscler Thromb Vasc Biol. 20:2175-2183, 2000.

Levonen, A. L., R. P. Patel, P. Brookes, Y. M. Go, H. Jo, S. Parthasarathy, P. G. Anderson, and V. M. Darley-Usmar. Mechanisms of cell signaling by nitric *oxide and peroxynitrite: from mitochondria to MAP kinases. Antioxid Redox Signal. 3:215-229, 2001.*

Lu, J., T. A. McKinsey, R. L. Nicol, and E. N. Olson. Signal-dependent activation of the MEF2 transcription factor by dissociation from histone deacetylases. Proc Natl Acad Sci U S A. 97:4070-4075, 2000.

Rao, G. N., N. R. Madamanchi, M. Lele, L. Gadiparthi, A. C. Gingras, T. E. Eling, and N. Sonenberg. A potential role for extracellular signal-regulated kinases in prostaglandin F2alpha-induced protein synthesis in smooth muscle cells. J Biol Chem. 274:12925-12932, 1999.

Trappe, T. A., F. White, C. P. Lambert, D. Cesar, M. Hellerstein, and W. J. Evans. Effect of ibuprofen and acetaminophen on postexercise muscle protein synthesis. Am J Physiol Endocrinol Metab. 282:E551-556, 2002.

Wilborn, C, M Roberts, C Kerksick, M Iosia, L Taylor, B Campbell, T Harvey, R Wilson, M. Greenwood, D Willoughby and R Kreider. Exercise & Sport Nutrition Laboratory, Center for Exercise, Nutrition & Preventive Health Research, Baylor University, Waco, TX 76798-7313.

8. **CLA** or Conjugated Linoleic Acid, is the controversial trans-fat. You can find your CLA in beef and dairy products, especially grass fed beef. The problem is that a lot of the time the CLA that is found in supplement form isn't the same chemically as natural CLA.

It's actually made from unhealthy vegetable oil most of the time. So, in my opinion I would either stay away from CLA as a supplement, or only get it from organic markets with very, very knowledgeable employees. With that said, it's great to get it from natural sources, which I am about to go into. The studies on CLA are very controversial.

There have been way too many studies

conducted on weight loss in rats and animals, so it's obvious that CLA causes weight loss in animals, but what about humans? There have been some studies on humans showing that people taking CLA vs. people taking a placebo lost a small percentage more weight over 12 weeks.

The problem that I have noticed time and time again is that we have no idea the differences in diet, or starting body composition of the people participating in the study. From my own research, I find that CLA studies in human subjects are leaning more towards the inconclusive side. Thus far, as practical fat loss goes, I wouldn't direct you to look towards CLA for fat loss, just look towards putting in the work.

I can't deny that it may make a 1% difference in fat loss, but I am all about bang for your buck and the amount of results you would hypothetically get from CLA is not worth the cost of the product in monetary value. Let's stick to natural sources of CLA. It seems that CLA, in some articles, makes you big and strong, and in other research and articles, makes you dead. Just like AA, I believe it's just another case of "helps bodybuilders but kills couch potatoes."

This stuff, like AA, is also found in meat and dairy so it makes sense, logically at least. It's really hard to find any hard pressed evidence of CLA being the super tablet that it's amped up to be in the fitness industry. I am sure that when you saw "CLA," you were ready to read about how amazing it is.

Sorry, I believe that getting enough CLA from natural beef and dairy products is great for people who live in an anabolic state, i.e. those of us who are weight training multiple days a week. CLA is a trans-fatty acid which is one of the reasons it's so controversial. It's very volatile, so trying to recreate it in supplement form is kind of like playing with fire.

I can't say anything for certain, but taking CLA in supplement form may do more bad than good. If you are a bodybuilder, or are looking to build a strong and powerful body, we can all conclude that beef and dairy are your friends, and they will help you build muscle.

This is the perfect example of why you should do your research on a supplement before going crazy on it, thinking it's going to get you shredded and help you build muscle. CLA is a form of Linoleic Acid, so it does have some of the same health benefits that other Linoleic Acids do. The thing is, there are tons of different forms of LA and they're all a little different. None of them can compare to the health benefits and awesomeness of ALA. This article is full of studies, take a look if you're interested.

9. **Lauric Acid** is the coolest saturated fat, ever. This is the medium chain Triglyceride (MCT) we talked about earlier that was found in coconut oil. Lauric Acid is a MCT that your body can easily absorb just as it would a carbohydrate.

   You can also find it in palm kernel oil. This is the MCT that is being studied to help people with developing mental conditions such as Alzheimer's.

The people of Tokelauans Island eat over 60% of their calories from coconuts and are the biggest consumers of saturated fat in the world.

Yes, you heard me, they are the biggest consumers of saturated fat in the world. What does this mean? Saturated fats aren't bad for you, nor all they all equal. Ironically, enough people that live on tropical Islands like the Tokelauans are some of the healthiest people in the world. They tend to be completely disease free, with no signs of heart disease anywhere. The high consumption of Lauric Acid in coconut oil does have something to do with this.

There are many other factors about a tropical diet, which we will go into in in Part 2. Lauric acid does actually have a fat burning affect because of the fact that it increases energy expenditure vs. other fat sources. By replacing your vegetable oils with coconut oil, you are doing yourself a favor in the long run. Just think about it, if you are losing weight and the calorie expense of coconut oil is just a little higher than say butter or olive oil, over time that's extra pounds lost because of one simple switch.

This stuff has been shown to increase calorie expenditure up to 5%, which is a lot! Consider this: if you are on a 2000 calorie diet, and eat a lot of coconut oil, you could easily be expending an extra 25 to 100 calories a day. Over a month, this adds up to .25 to 1 extra pound of body fat that you could be losing based on a 2,000 calorie diet. Yes, coconut oil is a thermogenic.

There was a study conducted at the Faculty of Medicine, University of Geneva. You know I am not big on studies, however I am a firm believer in the power of lauric acid and coconut oil. This study concluded that eating just 15 to 30 grams of coconut oil per day as a way to get lauric acid, literally increased calorie expenditure by 5%.

Now, we can always argue the relevance of any study, but there is so much supporting evidence that MCT's, lauric acid and coconut oil do amazing things, that I fully believe this. But how do you put this into practice? Simple, replace your olive oils, or any other vegetable oils with coconut oil or find another chunk of fat you can eliminate from your daily diet so that you can add a little coconut oil in its place.

Oh, and definitely replace butter with coconut oil, getting used to the taste is worth the super effects it has over butter. Coconut oil/ lauric acid has also been shown to reduce appetite, I can personally confirm this one though my own experiences. When supplementing with coconut oil, I tend to have less cravings and less of those sudden bursts of hunger throughout the day.

The thing is, anything that can reduce our appetite can be helpful. So if you're leaning down, or just looking to maintain a lean physique year around like most of us, lauric acid from coconut oil is your friend. As bodybuilders and fitness enthusiasts, it's easy to get really hung up on counting calories and macros. It's really easy to become obsessed with the numbers. Personally,

I believe that the discipline aspect of counting macros is great, you learn a lot about food, and you grow as a person.

The issue is that none of us should be counting calories 24/7/365. There are more important things in life than your food intake. We should learn macros, not marry them. If you are eating less calories per day without actively having to make that happen, you are winning in life.

This is like having your cake and eating it too, you're creating a larger calorie deficit without thinking about it, this is what will keep you lean year-round. It has been proven time and time again that the amount of calories you reduce from eating coconut oil as a result of its appetite-suppressing effects, range anywhere between 100 to 250 calories per day.

As far as fat burning goes, lauric acid and coconut oil are a double whammy. Not only is this fatty acid a thermogenic, but it's also a powerful appetite suppressant. So, in theory if you wanted to take the best of the best in terms of results in fat loss, you could be burning up to 400 more calories per day.

That is an extreme case, but my point is that it's pretty epic. No fat loss supplement that I know of can do that and be healthy at the same time. The only thing close to having anywhere near that size of calorie pool created by a thermogenic, would be an appetite suppressant/fat burner cocktail like those found in most fat burning pills. Only those would make you feel like you're dying all day.

Yet coconut oil does it and fights cancer and fuels the brain at the same time. This stuff may even become a cure for Alzheimer's in the future, that is a possibility. It also works well as a sunscreen, blocking nearly 20% of the sun's ultraviolet rays. It is also used to improve hair and keep the skin moist and healthy.

Oh, and it lowers LDL cholesterol and increases HDL. Need I say more? I would keep going and explain the science behind its thermogenic effects, appetite suppressant effects, health benefits, etc. but this book wasn't written to give you a chemistry lesson. Just take my word for it, lauric acid, MCT's, and coconut oil are the shit. Here is a link to an article with tons of linked scientific studies if you want to check them out.

10. **Fatclusion** There are tons of different fatty acids that do different things. Fats are, in my opinion, the most misunderstood macronutrient. The body can't go without essential fatty acids or it will slowly break down. Fats are a very big part of brain function and overall health, as well as muscular development.

Every fatty acid has some specific abilities, and some are much more valuable than others. My two favorite fatty acids in terms of bang for your buck, are ALA and lauric acid, as you can probably tell. Those two fatty acids provide an insane amount of health, muscle building and fat burning benefits.

Understanding why things work and also why other things are bullshit is very valuable information for anyone looking to become bigger, leaner, stronger, heathier, happier and more confident. It's crucial to understand fat down to the individual fatty acid level so that in Part 2 of the book, you understand where I am coming from when talking about different diets and which one may be best for you, or even why a mix of several diets may be ideal.

Fats do everything from regulating your blood pressure to preventing mental illnesses, to building muscle and burning fat, and you can't live without them. Now that you understand fat, carb and protein, we can now look into different ways of eating using them.

Sit back, relax and take this in. This book contains everything you need to become efficient and effective with your food lifestyle a/k/a dieting. But remember, I only use the word "diet" because it is the practical term when talking about eating lifestyle, healthy lifestyle, etc.

The truth is, there is no one diet, this is not something you will do overnight, or over a month, and this book is the modern day guide on how to change your habitual eating habits.

This book is for those who want to become elite, bigger, stronger, more powerful, abnormally healthy, happy, and confident. This book is not for the dabbler, it's for those of us who want to make things happen. If you are serious about your health and physique, keep reading.

If you are just dabbling and bullshitting yourself and everyone around you, listen to what I am about to say. You love to eat up all of the marketing bullshit, eat this superfood, lose 30 pounds in 30 days with this fat burning supplement, build 20 pounds of muscle in just one month by eating this way. You, my friend, are a headline reader and you're not going to do shit but keep buying things that promise great value only to find out the same thing over and over again.

There are tons of different ways to do things, but you should be looking for the shiny object in the room that promises super human results. You need to understand the basic fundamentals, and then here's the important part: stop being a lazy shithead and go put the things in this book into practice and build a physique that you can be proud of.

It's hard to break a habitually lazy mind, and habitually lazy will power - and you may think that I am being hard on you and that I'm an asshole. Here's the thing, the rest of your life will be ten times better if you choose today to break out of your habitual thinking and go make shit happen. If you are already in that mindset, "My Man", LET'S GO MAKE SOME GAINZ!

SECTION 2

THE 3 FORMS OF DIETING

Throw What You Know Out the Window.

Most of the things we learn about dieting, meal frequency and meal timing are irrelevant in practical application. Take a deep breath; I am about to debunk a lot of myths right now.

- There is no optimal meal frequency
- No optimal meal timing
- No optimal amount of protein
- No optimal amount of fat
- No optimal amount of carbs

- There is no 30-minute anabolic window post workout
- Not eating breakfast isn't bad, in fact I do it
- Intermittent fasting doesn't yield super fat loss abilities
- Eating food before bed doesn't make you store fat
- Keto diets with no carbs don't provide you with super fat burning abilities
- An absurd amount of protein every day won't help you build more muscle
- All processed foods aren't bad
- All natural foods aren't good
- Dieting isn't hard, following a healthy lifestyle is not hard
- You can lose weight eating a lot of carbs
- Saturated fat is not bad
- You can get shredded eating at McDonalds daily
- You can look good, feel good and perform well all while eating delicious foods that you enjoy.
- You can eat the amount of meals you want to eat, at the time you want to eat them and get the results you want to have. The best part is that it's not hard or complicated.
- The tooth fairy isn't real, and no, pigs don't fly, silly marketers.

Find a Way of Eating That Works for You.

The point I am trying to make here is that dieting, or eating in a way that leads you to your goals short-term and long-term, is not hard. There is no special diet that gives everyone results; you can get in shape on any "diet." The eating protocol you should follow is the eating protocol that you will enjoy and adhere to.

Effectiveness and efficiency do not mean a damn thing if you hate the diet protocol. Enduring a diet you don't like may yield some great short term results, but in the long run, will hurt you much more than help you.

If you're struggling to adhere to a diet protocol you hate, that you wanted to quit before you even started, you're hurting yourself in the long run. When you have a bad experience with a way of dieting, i.e. eating to achieve a particular objective that requires eating in a way that doesn't align with your lifestyle, the foods you like, and it doesn't make you happy - don't do it.

Building a diet around what you like to eat, and when you like to eat is so much more important than doing the diet that is "at this moment in time" marketed to get you results. For a way of eating to help your relationship with food and not hurt it, your new way of eating needs to be a couple of things. First of all, it needs to be something that compliments your life and doesn't stress you out.

The second thing is it needs to be a diet that involves a meal frequency and a meal timing that coincides with your lifestyle and doesn't contradict it. Third, it needs to be a diet that is an easy transition from the way you are already eating. Whatever restaurants you are habitually eating at, don't cut them all out. If you are already eating at Chipotle, just change up your burrito a little, drop the cheese and sour cream. If you eat at Wendy's, get their fresh chicken sandwich or try their salad.

I could keep giving you examples, but the point is dieting is not what society makes it out to be. If you are on the opposite side of the coin and you're struggling to gain weight and build muscle, just do the opposite. Take what you are already eating and add more, or add more of the foods you like, slowly increase calories. You're bulking, bulking is fun.

There is also the performance and feel good side of this. Some people do better with high carb diets, some people do better with high fat diets, and some people do better on a paleo diet. I know people that enjoy eating every couple of hours and I know people that would much rather eat a feast once or twice a day.

Personally, I enjoy 3 meals a day. Some people enjoy counting their macronutrients, this is my favorite approach and a method of manipulating calories that I prefer, but it's not for everybody. It seems the people that enjoy flexible dieting hate meal plans. On the contrary, the people that do better on meal plans hate flexible dieting.

There are even some people that hate meal plans *and* flexible dieting. For these people, intuitive dieting is the best way of going about eating, by making some changes in daily food choices every week, and eating sparingly only until full.

Then there is the third part of this dieting puzzle: are you trying to bulk up and build muscle, lose some body fat, get shredded for a bodybuilding show or go on a lean bulking phase? I will say that it's very difficult to get show ready using intuitive eating, but equally unnecessary to count macros to go on a small mini cut. And its blatant sabotage to be on a meal plan when bulking unless you're a top class IFBB pro bodybuilder.

I could put one client on flexible dieting using 300 carbs, 150 protein and 60 fat and get him shredded, and have another client that uses these macros as bulking macros, and then another client that will never even pay attention to the numbers and just wants a set meal plan.

I may have one client that looks and performs better on a fat based keto diet and another client that does much better on a high carb diet. It's not complicated, the important thing to take from what I am saying is that any diet will work for about anyone short term, but the goal is to find an eating protocol that you can marry and not one that's just a one-night stand.

In this Chapter, I'm going to be explaining in detail the three general eating protocols. These are not set in stone and I'm not saying you have to adopt one over another. My main goal is to give you the information you need so you can choose what's best for you.

The three protocols are:

- Flexible Dieting (or IIFYM/If it fits your macros), which involves tracking your macros in a way that maximizes your life and diet while giving you some wiggle room.

- Intuitive Eating (or I.E.), which encourages the development of a healthy relationship between you and your food.

- Meal Plans (Bro Diet), which represent a structured way of getting in your exact macronutrients while embracing a 'set it and forget it' philosophy.

All three of these types of diets have extensive benefits and some drawbacks. Keep reading to gain a complete understanding of each of them so you can move ahead with the food lifestyle that's perfect for you.

Flexible Dieting/ IIFYM (If it fits your macros)

Let me just start by saying flexible dieting is the most commonly misunderstood methods of dieting on the face of the earth. Not only is it misunderstood by most, it is also used a lot of the time to justify eating a majority of daily calories from shit "because it fits your macros."

Flexible dieting is very controversial; some people swear by it, and others crucify it. I believe it is great for many reasons. First of all, we established that we can eat whatever we want and still lose weight and build muscle. Secondly, it made dieting ten times easier for some individuals that just don't take well to meal plans. Thirdly is the fact that it's much more accurate than many other forms of dieting, which is great for people who are serious about keeping a certain body fat year-round or achieving sub 10% body fat.

Flexible dieting is even a great dieting protocol to follow when in a lean bulk phase because it allows you to eat what you want while maintaining a lean physique. Someone people have no control in a bulking phase and need some structure.

Before IIFYM, you would typically see bodybuilders eating nothing but rice, sweet potatoes, and oats for weight loss and building muscle. Why did we eat so selectively? Because eating simple sugars made our blood sugar rise and making our blood sugar rise directly caused our pancreas to release insulin, which in turn resulted in fat gain.

From what you read in the first section, and the data

we now know, this is not the case. Guys, gaining fat has little to do with just one hormonal response. Fat gain comes from a habitual surplus of calories. As far as losing fat loss or muscle gain is concerned, a carb is a carb.

What I am saying is you could lose the same amount of weight using doughnuts and pop tarts as your carb source as sweet potatoes and rice. At this point, any bro scientist would blow up and blurt out all of the bullshit studies he read in said magazine the somehow proved IIFYM to be untrue.

The problem is, you can eat shit and get ripped, and it's been scientifically proven through the laws of thermodynamics. The thing is, that's not flexible dieting, that's molested flexible dieting. It's called "flexible dieting" because it's flexible. Let me give you an example.

Flexible dieting is predicated off of hitting your target fat, carb, and protein numbers every day as well as fiber and micronutrients. Let's say your macros are 60 fat, 300 carb, and 180 protein. You eat 4 meals a day; you get 2-4 servings of vegetables per day and 1-3 servings of fruit, your diet is based mostly on nutrient-dense complex carbs, high quality omega-3, omega-6 and saturated fats, and your protein sources are based off of high BV sources of protein.

At the end of the day, if you have 30 carbs, 12 grams of fat, and 7 grams of protein left over, and that will allow you to fit one doughnut into your macros at the end of the day, go for it, it's not cheating. Don't think of it as cheating, you fit it in perfectly. Please keep in mind this is just an example of eating whatever you want. But if you're fitting in processed food with HFCS and Trans-fat all day, eventually it's going to catch up to you.

In my opinion, the diet plan guys that think all flexible

dieters eat shit all day are wrong, and the flexible dieters who think all meal plan guys are "bros" are also wrong. We are all on the same side, we are all gym obsessed, food obsessed weirdos. Besides, from a subjective point of view, a meal plan, or any other type of diet is still counting macros. You're still fitting in macros, just with a much narrower selection of food choices and sometimes food timing guidelines.

Most flexible dieters use a little macro counting app called "MyFitnessPal" and it works shockingly well. For instance, all you need to do to enter that crispy crème doughnut into your macros for the day is open the app and search the food item in the food database, boom - "plain doughnut from Krispy Crème" = 11 fat, 21 carb, 2 protein with 1 gram of fiber. One cup of brown rice (minute made) cooked is 2.2 fat, 51 carb, 4.5 protein and 3 grams of fiber.

Once you enter the numbers into your macros for the day, you know how many macros you have just spent out of your daily quota and you also know how many macros you have left. This works with anything with a barcode, any fruit or vegetable, any restaurant, etc. Flexible dieting when done right is a beautiful thing.

I recommend it if you are craving some sort of food item one day or have a date that night, to plan for it; be sparing with your macros that day and if you want something, eat it. Going about dieting this way makes life easier. If you want to go out with the BAE and get steak and wine, go for it. If you can split a dessert and still not go over your macros, enjoy it my friend. But be leery, the lower your macros become when dieting to get lean, the less you want to try fitting things in.

If you're only at 35 fat and 200 carb, you shouldn't

be fitting in 2 pop tarts. On the contrary, if you are eating 500 carbs and 80 fat, you can fit in different things. There are tons of great ways to make your entire diet fun when counting macros, like low sugar syrup, low sugar sauces, low sugar ketchup, bbq sauce, etc. You would be surprised at how easy it is to eat this way, counting macros, once you get used to it.

Flexible Dieting is an Education

When it comes to dieting, not everyone needs to diet using the molecular breakdown of fat, protein and carbs. But understanding food and thermodynamics is crucial for anyone looking to develop a physique.

A lot of us grew into the fitness industry thinking we needed only complex carbs and super high protein to build muscle and burn fat. This couldn't possibly be further from the truth. For the newbies out there, it's important to learn the basic fundamental truth. The body will burn fat on a caloric deficit, which is burning more than you take in. Your body will maintain body composition on a caloric maintenance, and your body will gain muscle on a caloric surplus.

If you're just beginning, for example you're new to lifting and new into eating to grow or eating to shred, it's important to understand these fundamentals. You have fat, carbs, and protein, and understanding how much you personally need of each per day to be on a deficit, maintenance, or surplus, is very important for your long-term success.

Diet plans are great, but they don't give you the deep understanding about your body and food that counting macros does. Your macro levels should be based on your gender, your lean body composition, your overall caloric intake and your bodyweight.

It would be really easy for me to spout out macro ratios, like your diet should compose of 58% carbs, 25% protein and 17% fat. Let's say a male bodybuilder is dieting on 3000 calories at 58% C, 25% P and 17% F, which would make his macros 435C, 188P, and 57F. Our male bodybuilder, let's call him Dick, is fairly active, 24 years old, 5 foot 7 and has a pretty strong basal metabolic rate. His starting bodyweight is 190lb and his goal with these macros is about 180lb bodyweight. He loses the first 7 pounds very easily because of water weight loss, because his bulking macros which were much higher. In about one month, he's down almost 8 pounds, still looking full.

At this point we can either up his macros, because he's losing weight fast, or ride them out another week or two. As a coach, I decide we should ride them out another week or two. We ride out another week and the scale only drops 1 pound, the next week we see .75. Now let me just say, this is perfect weight loss, 75% of weight loss won't be this straight forward.

After 6 weeks on these macros, he is starting to really slow down, so if we would have upped the macros 2 weeks ago, it would have netted us a loss of time in terms of weight loss, which is fine if you don't have a due date to be lean by. But if you do, moving forward as smoothly as possible is the goal.

Once weight loss subsides to less than .5 pounds lost per week or less, it's time to make some changes. The body has fully adapted to this calorie level, and now, in order to pull off more body fat, we must either drop carbs, drop fat or add in some cardio.

The choice can vary greatly depending on the coach, the athlete, the situation and the preferences of both coach and athlete. Let's say in this case I lower Dick's carbs to 405. Personally, in the first quarter of a lean down phase, I like to lower carbs; cardio would come later, and the third action would be to lower fat.

I like to keep fat up as long as possible for many reasons, and keep cardio down as long as possible since the goal is to lift weights. I would prefer most of the athlete's calories to be burned by having an intense workout.

On top of that, cardio takes more time and requires more time management, especially when most people have jobs and families. Now as this goes on, the athlete is learning about their body. They now know, ok at 190, I can lose weight at 3000 calories, or 435C, 188P and 57F, relatively easily. They also know at 180 that changes will need to be made. This is why I say that counting macros is an education.

Flexible dieting is a low priced, super high value, effective and efficient education. I actually was coached for about a year by Jeff Alberts of Team 3DMJ, and after 10 years of doing this stuff myself, I started taking on clients and I still do. Now, you don't need a coach, but sometimes having a subjective point of view, and someone who has done this for a long time behind you, is a good idea.

If you find the right coach, it's a highly underpriced service for the value. Here is the thing; these macro ratios may work great for a 190-pound male bodybuilder with a great BMR at the age of 24, but what about Lisa? Yep, I just went there. Let's say Lisa is a 35-year-old mom with little free time, a much slower BMR, and is someone who just wants to get lean for a before and after transformation, not a physique comp.

Not everybody wants to have some elaborate competition. A lot of people, maybe even you, just want to show the world what you can do. Lisa is starting out at 115lbs and just wants to get a leaner, tighter look, a "fit mom transformation." By nature, the amount of calories you burn will be directly related to your bodyweight, so someone weighing 115 is going to burn much less calories than someone at 190.

Also, women have a harder time losing weight than men because of how their hormones react to weight loss. In order for Lisa to lose weight, her calories need to be at about 1800 with 58%C, 25%P, 17%F, which would put little Lisa at 261C, 113P, and 34F. Those aren't bad numbers, but I would like to see a little more fat, and I don't think Lisa needs that much protein because her lean body mass is much less than 113lbs.

What I would want to start Lisa on is 55%C, 23%P, and 24%F. We would be looking at 245C, 104P, and 48F. These are much better macros in my opinion. I don't like to see them get too low and I don't think there is any need for a crap ton of protein. Of course this very hugely varies on a person by person basis. I do believe that women need to make sure to get enough fats because their hormones are so much more volatile than in men.

So Lisa starts out and after her first month, loses 3 pounds. Doesn't sound like much, but for a 115-pound woman, that's phenomenal. That would even be good weight loss for someone starting at 150. Going into month two, weight loss stops completely. Now we need to make a change. Let's take the carbs down to 230.

Now we are back to around .5 pounds lost per week.

The good thing is we have some balanced macros to play with moving forward and we aren't doing much physical activity yet, so if we need to add in a cardio session or even drop fat, we can do it.

As Lisa moves forward, I would keep things the same as long as possible until we hit another weight loss plateau. Once we hit another plateau, I would drop carbs to 215 and keep it moving. At this point we should net some good weight loss and get closer to that desired after-look. Since we have lowered carbs twice, my next move would be to add in a little more physical activity for Lisa, not too much though, balance is key. This may get us all the way to our goal. If not, we have a lot of wiggle room with the fats.

Dropping fat is the last thing I will do, but dropping to 40 fat could mean hitting the goal. The beautiful thing is that both Lisa and Dick now understand their body much better than they did before counting macros, and since it's flexible dieting, they weren't tied down to any specific food choices.

Understanding that macros are completely different from person to person is key. You may not be able to eat like an IFBB pro bodybuilder and get lean, and a 115-pound woman won't be able to eat like you and get lean. It's a learning process, and an education.

Misconceptions about IIFYM

As I stated earlier, a lot of people like to point the finger at flexible dieters and say, "you guys eat nothing but pop tarts and doughnuts." When IIFYM became popular, it became a trend to fit pop tarts and Chipotle into your macros.

The entirety of this trend, or the whole point, was to show that dieting can be fun - you can fit in less nutritious foods sparingly when you get the craving. When you fit in foods that you want when you get cravings, it makes an eating protocol ten times easier to follow in the long run.

When we are still able to go out with friends and eat out at Chipotle post workout, have a steak dinner at Longhorn Steakhouse, or have a 2am breakfast at IHOP and still get into great shape, that's what makes IIFYM as a protocol, revolutionary. It is the diet that makes sense because it isn't restrictive; you don't need to eat seven times a day and you can be a somewhat normal human being and an athlete at the same time.

There are some people who will use the methods and guidelines of flexible dieting and still eat 100% nutrient dense foods 99% of the time. And there are those other people that will fit 3 slices of pizza and 2 doughnuts into their macros every day. Neither of them are wrong for the way they diet, I could argue both sides. I could argue pizza doughnut guy is probably eating too much shit, but I could also argue that 99% guy is a complete bro and doesn't enjoy life.

There will always be a divide: the 100% clean eaters will say that pizza doughnut guys are terrible people because blah blah blah, and the pizza doughnut guy will say that the 100% clean eaters are "bros" and will assume they're stupid.

It's completely up to you to dictate what is right and wrong in your head. Everyone has their own idea of what is acceptable in the dieting and nutrition world. I myself just don't like extremes, period. Fitting a bunch of processed shit into your macros, in my opinion, is hurting you in the long run.

Remember the first section of the book where I broke down fat, carbs, and protein to their molecular levels? Well, in terms of immediate weight loss or weight gain, a carb is a carb. The whole "a calorie is a calorie" statement is probably the worst statement in the diet industry, whether you are trying to say it's true or false. That statement is more dependent on context than a high school girl is dependent on attention.

In terms of weight loss or weight gain on a macro level, from a 'loss' perspective, a calorie is a calorie, granted your comparing carbs to carbs, fats to fats, and proteins to proteins. On a slightly below the surface area, no, a calorie is not a calorie, and no, a carb is not a carb. There are millions of different molecularly structured carbs, fats and proteins.

Take the macros for example – 200 protein, 400 carb, 65 fat. From a base level above ground look, if you're hitting these macros, you are hitting these macros, but the sources of these macros makes no difference in terms of short term fat loss.

Here is the thing, from my first chapter you know that different proteins have different levels of biological value, no BV isn't bro science, it's a fact. If all of your carbs were from refined foods, mostly from HFCS, and all of your fats were from fried foods and hydrogenated oils with trans-fatty acids, wouldn't you still be hitting your macros? Yes, you would but that is molesting IIFYM.

You may get shredded but you may also lose muscle and die in the process if you're susceptible to any sort of health conditions whatsoever, like every human on the planet.

Granted, some people can eat like this and be fine, but I don't recommend it for anybody. The other guy gets his protein from "Whey Hydroslate," which is chemically altered to have the highest BV of any form of protein. He also strategically adds in other high BV sources of protein like eggs and fish. He makes sure to eat all of his carbs from complex carbs sources, high nutrient veggies and fruits. He also makes sure to take both omega-3 fatty acids in supplement form, as well as ALA separately, and some omega-6, and 1 tablespoon of coconut oil.

He also makes sure to get a variety of fish in every day for natural sources of essential fatty acids. He even goes so far as to take BCAA's intro workout and take Beta-Alanine, L-Arginine pre workout along with his pre workout concoction. Damn money bags, this guy is probably spending $800 a month on food and supplementation easily. The other guy could be under $300 a month.

These are two opposite extremes. I don't think you should eat pop tarts and pizza all day with Quest Protein Chips as your protein sources, but there is also no reason to spend your entire life trying to be perfect, it's not that big of a deal.

I like the human approach, eat 80-90% nutrient dense food, high BV protein like basic whey, eggs and chicken, get your omega-3 and omega-6 fatty acids through a little fish or supplementation, and get at least 2 to 3 servings of green veggies, 1-3 servings of fruit, and 2-4 servings of complex carbs.

Also make sure to hit your fiber at around 1 gram per 100 calories. If you have room to fit in a doughnut or a slice of pizza, go for it "in moderation." At the end of the day, genes also play a part, so does metabolism, muscle density, etc. I know a guy who weighs 167 and deadlifts more than me who is perfectly healthy. He eats about 6,000 calories a day, drinks 2 liters of diet soda, and eats pizza and candy, even a whole container of ice-cream. He maintains his 160 bodyweight and deadlifts nearly 600 pounds. He has no signs of bad health.

Personally, I would become obese, diabetic, go into a depression and probably eventually die doing this. I know others who eat nothing but complex carbs, high BV proteins and high quality fats that are also super healthy, jacked, ripped and strong. It all comes down to you: every single person in the world has a very different body chemistry for millions of different reasons.

We must not base our methods on what anyone else does because we are all very different in practice. IIFYM can be molded to anyone, this is why it is so insanely popular. IIFYM is more of a practical macro template than an actual diet protocol, and flexible dieting is what you make of it.

Flexible Dieting/IIFYM Cons

It's not for everyone. There are different types of cons to flexible dieting, cons that I didn't mention earlier. This way of eating isn't perfect, and for people that don't mesh well with flexible dieting, it may be bad for their lifestyle and their psychology. These are the different reasons and different types of people that may not mesh with IIFYM.

- If you are someone who doesn't like counting things and you don't like putting numbers on activities, you will not like IIFYM and it will not work for you. Sometimes it can be a daunting task to make sure you hit your numbers for fat, carb and protein every day. It's an obligation, another task you must meet.

  Counting macros may be that one thing

that overwhelms some people. Think about it, everything you eat has to be tracked. If your diet is super diverse in food variety, food portions, food timing, etc., counting macros does take a little work to stay on top of it.

If you're eating a large salad with ten different ingredients, have a nice time trying to track all of that. If you are making a shake with fruits, veggies, protein and oils, you're going to be mentally drained trying to track that.

Here is what I will say to those people who like to make extravagant meals, and who also want to utilize IIFYM as their dieting protocol: build your perfect salad with the portion sizes you want in it and build the meal using the MyFitnessPal app. Call your salad the "insert your name here" salad. For example, there is a shredded YouTuber that makes his own salads, massive salads every night, and even mixes a Chipotle bowl in. You may know him, his name is Matt Ogus, pretty cool guy and one who helped put eating giant salads and Chipotle on the map, regarding IIFYM at least. You can do the same things with your precious monster nutrition shakes.

- Another potential downfall of IIFYM is the fact that it can be a serious health food deterrent. It was never meant to be a health food deterrent, go figure. Since the IIFYM diet is predicated on numbers, you "could" hypothetically fit nothing but refined, processed, molested foods into your diet.

The sad thing is that a large portion of flexible dieters use it for exactly that, to justify eating shit all day. If you are someone who is looking for any possible reason to eat like crap all of the time and justify it, don't take up flexible dieting. You my friend probably need a meal plan, or you need to go sit in the corner and have time out.

IIFYM is not a justification for eating crap all day, it's simply a method of tracking what you eat in order to get leaner, build muscle or educate yourself on your body's macro needs. A lot of people are just lazy, yep I said it, and you may be too lazy for IIFYM. If counting what you eat all day makes you hate life, then you probably should find another way to hit your goals.

Sometimes it can get just plain annoying when it's the end of the day and you are left with some weird macros like 30 protein, 2 fat and 31 carbs. Yep, time to become a mathematician because of IIFYM. To avoid this happening to you, plan for that last meal, save some fat and carbs so you can enjoy yourself later in the evening or before bed.

Stick to protein earlier in the day and be sparing with your fat and carbs so that you can fit that cookie in while studying for your exam tonight, or while you watch Netflix and chill. Yep, no need to act like a crazed dieting mixologist in front of your Netflix and chill date. Save yourself and have those fat and carb macros waiting for you that fateful night.

- If you're a dieting perfectionist, tread lightly with IIFYM, maybe you should just walk away. Trying to hit your macro numbers perfectly may actually turn your brain cells into computer storage, and you may start doing the robot, because you may be becoming a robot and nobody likes robots.

There is absolutely no reason to need to be exact on your macro numbers at the end of the day. If your numbers are 55F, 225C, 155P and at the end of the day you were at 53F, 220C, 151P, you will be perfectly fine if you don't go take baby bites of chicken and eat a blueberry with 2 grams of peanut butter. I followed strict macros for one full year of my bodybuilding career, and for almost that entire year I did not break my macros. Shit, I even had bad dreams about breaking my macros by 20 grams or so.

Seriously, I had bad dreams about hurting my precious macros. The point is, don't be obsessed with hitting your numbers perfectly. If you go over by 25 grams on carbs one day, and it's not a refeed day, it isn't the end of the world. The whole macro breaking self-shaming thing doesn't do anything but hurt you and make you want to stop counting macros.

Another thing that you will notice, which is equally as good for some individuals as it is bad for others, is that you will always feel obligated to finish your food. The problem with this is that over time, psychologically, this primes you to always finish your food.

If you never finish your food and constantly under eat, this reprogramming of the cognitive habitual eating habits is a good thing. However, if you tend to have a bad relationship with food and always finish food, but the meals you are finishing involve way too much food, this may just put the nail in the coffin for an overeating eating disorder. If you have an eating disorder, you have to really tread carefully on your eating habits.

Different diet protocols can even create potential eating disorders. Wiring yourself to always finish your food can turn into always finishing a pizza, or always finishing a box of doughnuts. I myself have this problem at the moment, which is why I am intuitive dieting until I feel as though my relationship with food is on par to go back to IIFYM.

The things is, it's different for everyone; some people need to finish their food because they never do, i.e. you ladies do this a lot. If your BF cooks your food, you better finish it, seriously, finish it. It's up to you to play it smart with dieting; your relationship to food is critical and much more important than your method of eating or dieting.

- For those who are going on a long-term bulk, IIFYM isn't necessary year-round. If you have been bulking for a while and you understand about the amount of food you need to eat to slowly gain weight, then there is no reason to strictly count macros, in my opinion.

If you are naturally very skinny or find it hard to gain weight at all, I don't see any pressing reason to count macros. When you're bulking, this should be your time to have fun; eat weird desserts that you aren't tracking macros for, have days where your fats may be a little higher or your carbs may be a little higher.

When you're deep into a bulk, have fun, this is your time to be less mindful of food. I am not saying get fat, I am saying eat food without thinking "I must track this food item for I must hit my macros." Personally, after I end a cutting/fat loss phase and transition into a lean bulking phase, I stay on macros for about 2 months, then I transition into intuitive eating, or eating until I'm comfortably full.

I just don't think we should be tracking macros year-round. I have no idea what's in that weird meal at that Japanese restaurant I ate at a couple of months ago, and I sure as hell wasn't going to track it into my macros.

- For individuals who are extremely overweight, and have hormones out of whack and need to just start eating better, IIFYM is absolutely not the way to go. If you are morbidly overweight, the last thing you need to be thinking about is fitting a doughnut into your macros.

I think as a whole, meaning as a society, we have gone really soft on obesity. It's not ok. When you are highly overweight, you are basically a drug addict to highly refined, calorie dense food, calorie dense snacks, and calorie dense drinks. Because of your addiction, your hormones are all out of whack.

What you need to do is learn how to eat until 80% full, not 120% full. You need to stop drinking calories. By this I mean whatever you're drinking that has calories, cut it down by 90% or stop drinking drinks with over 50 calories period. You also need to cut out all refined, processed foods, cut down on breads, even whole grain breads. You need to cut down on any refined foods with HFCS, cut out butter and replace it with coconut oil.

Pay attention to food labels. Fill your diet with mainly green veggies and leaves like spinach and lettuce. Consume lean sources of protein like grilled chicken breast, fatty fishes, lean beef, eggs and whey protein. Eat highly nutritious complex carbs like sweet potatoes, brown rice, quinoa and plain oatmeal. Make sure to eat a couple servings of fruit every day, diversity is good – apples, blueberries, raspberries, bananas, grapes, etc. I have just solved your obesity problem.

Once you get used to making better food choices, and have a great relationship with healthy natural food, then you can try to dial in your dieting methods and protocol. Until then, IIFYM is not a good idea. A person who is addicted to drugs shouldn't be rewarded with drugs just because it's not enough drugs to hurt them at the end of the day if it fits in their macros.

- IIFYM is slightly more difficult when traveling, or eating out often. The problem when eating out is that you're never really 100% sure about what portion sizes are going to come out for your food. It's not that bad, but at the same time you will be more food focused if you're eating out a lot and counting macros.

- Since your food probably has extra cooking oil in it, accuracy is far from ideal when eating out. Here is what I say to people who are eating out and trying to get shredded at the same time: ask the restaurants not to use butter for cooking, get your veggies steamed, ask for the sauces for your foods on the side, get the same meal every time and be consistent at the restaurant.

Dieting with macros is much easier if you have a little structure in what you eat every week. You would probably do it anyway. When you're traveling, it's much easier to want to just snack all day. You tend to just eat what's available when traveling. It can be like a scavenger hunt on Easter day when traveling and trying to find your macros in the hotel café.

Not only will it be a lot of fun hunting to fit your macros, you will also spend all of your money on the $7 protein shakes and the $8 sub that the hotel café offers. It's almost as if hotels plot against flexible dieters. IIFYM could be a big money maker for destination hotels, think about it.

Here's how to avoid this potential IIFYM headache - bring a jug of your favorite protein with you, also bring a small portable blender. When you touch down at your traveling locations/ checkpoints, find your local Walmart and go get your essentials for IIFYM survival. It's really essential for an IIFYM traveler to have a go-to carb source, protein source, and fat source. For me, I bring a bucket of tasty whey protein, purchase some coconut milk, a bag of apples, a bag of spinach leaves, a box of brown or basmati rice, a glass container of coconut oil plus a few jugs of water.

Get your list ready beforehand and you will save your wallet and your physique. Really, this is advice you can take on any diet, but I will tell you this, if you're traveling, it's in your best interest to be a flexible dieter or intuitive eater (meal plans are hell when traveling). It is possible to stay on top of your diet and training while traveling. It just takes a little planning and preparation.

Flexible Dieting/IIFYM Pros

Flexible dieting is one of the best forms of dieting in my opinion because it's very versatile and much more fun than a meal plan, yet has structure in numbers which gives it the potential to be one of the most accurate forms of eating/dieting.

- If you are the type of person that needs a little structure in your diet, but isn't into having a set meal plan, flexible dieting is for you. You are the type of person who wants their cake and wants to eat it, too. You are the type of person who wants to look good aesthetically and also wants to be abnormally strong for your bodyweight.

   You want to have a structure that can shift in any direction that is needed in the moment; you want to be the sky scraper that sways with the wind. You're the type of person that has things that need to get done every day, every week, and every month, but you're flexible on when that happens. 100% structure makes you sad.

   I salute you because I, my friend, can completely relate to you. In fact, this is me as well.

Sometimes it's nice to save all of your fat and carb macros for that nice dinner date; other times you want to go blow half of your macros on Sunday breakfast at IHOP.

Sometimes it's really nice to have that big cookie with a tall coffee at the coffee shop. There will be days where you just want to be rebellious and eat crap. If you do that every once in a while, IIFYM will permit it. There may be days and weeks where you want to structure your macros like a meal plan, you can do that too.

• Refeed days - are those days where you get to eat a few extra carbs. Let me explain; you will be dropping your fat a little, and you could even drop your protein a little and up your carbs. This gives you a day to refuel your mind and body. For example, let's say your macros are 65F, 300C, 200P. On a refeed day you could drop the fat to 55 grams, drop the protein to 180 and up the carbs to 400 grams.

This way, on refeed day, you have a little more room to play, a mental break from your set macros, a day for you to feel more full, a day for you to purposely overreach on your macros without feeling bad about it. Now, that is one way to have a refeed - upping carbs and dropping fat and protein a little.

This is the type of refeed that most people use when on IIFYM, especially contest preppers. They really need that buffer day for several reasons. There are other ways to refeed, too. If you like eating higher fat foods, you can drop the protein in favor of more fat on your refeed day, or up the carbs and protein a little bit.

The great thing is that you aren't cheating yourself, or IIFYM, you're sticking to a macro protocol. You can't do this with meal plans because, well, you aren't counting the macros plus you have to stick to certain foods. If you eat something out of your meal plan, "you're cheating." Just the thought of cheating on a diet, just that word "cheating," is bad news.

If you are shaming yourself for cheating on your diet, chances are you will start to develop some self-hatred for the so called cheating on your diet. The problem is, you're hating yourself for being a normal human with normal cravings. Hardcore classic dieters will say that refeeding is cheating, I say that they are stupid.

- There is no cheating with IIFYM, there is only fitting. It's very well known that trying to suppress cravings for a certain food will only lead to the obsession of those foods and the urge to want to binge on them.

It's the reverse psychology effect; telling yourself you can't have something creates an eagerness inside you until eventually, you have that which you can't have in the moment. We want what we can't have, it's human nature, its psychology 101. Why do you think we have Oreo, waffle, and birthday cake flavored whey protein? If you want an Oreo cookie, eat a fucking Oreo cookie.

I myself am a cookie monster; I have learned

to accept that about myself. Instead of trying to tell myself I am not a cookie monster, I simply fit a cookie into my diet almost every day.

Ironically, when you're following flexible dieting, just knowing you can fit whatever you want into your diet reduces your cravings down to something that is manageable. You don't have to wait 12 weeks to eat pizza and ice-cream, you can eat them now and guess what? You can eat that pizza and ice-cream now, and still lose weight.

Just don't turn what I am saying into the reason you fit a bunch of shit into your diet every single day because you read it in this book, because I am not saying that. What I am saying is, if you want to experience taco Tuesday this week, do it, if you want Chipotle for dinner, do it, if you want a doughnut pre workout tomorrow, do it. Are you starting to see the appeal of flexible dieting?

• You can fit alcohol in your macros. Alcohol is its own macro, so plan for that one beer you want to have with your buddies later, or 2, whatever floats your boat. Don't go crazy and get drunk, that not good for getting shredded or building muscle.

What you can do is if you want to have a couple of beers one evening drop some carbs and trade them in for some alcohols. Let's say you want to drink two beers that are 100 calories a piece; save 50 carbs for those 2 beers, there you go you party animal. Try to stay under 3 beers; remember, too much alcohol can affect fat loss and muscle gain because your body has a hard time ridding itself of alcohol.

- Diet breaks are easier with IIFYM, as compared with intuitive eating and meal plans, which are discussed in detail after this section. If you are an athlete of any kind, like a bodybuilder or a physique competitor, or if you do photoshoots displaying your physique, whenever you diet for any long period of time, diet breaks are very necessary. If you are on a caloric deficit longer than 20 weeks, I recommend you look into diet breaks.

I personally have been on caloric deficits 30 weeks + and I don't recommend this for anyone under 20% body fat. Now, if you are dieting down and losing 100 pounds or more, you would probably be ok, although diet breaks would still be very useful for you as well.

The thing is, a diet break can either be a good thing, or a bad thing. If you just go crazy and stuff your face for a week on a diet break, you could potentially destroy "in one week" what it took you months and months to diet down to.

In some cases, I have seen people go off of a diet and gain every bit of weight lost over a year back in a little over a week. Yes, it's possible, and not hard to do. When we are on a caloric deficit for a long period of time and are relatively low in body fat, leptin levels drop down. Leptin is the hormone responsible for telling your brain that you are full. The longer you stay on a caloric deficit the more this hormone will drop.

When leptin levels get really low, you stay hungry all of the time, it feels like you are always starving. You could binge eat, and you still wouldn't feel satisfied, just sad. One way to buffer the drop of leptin levels is scheduled refeeds. When dieting long-term, a 1-week diet break can be crucial every 16-20 weeks in order to not get depressed, not want to binge, keep a somewhat healthy relationship with food, bring hormones back up, give the CNS a rest, etc.

The way I like to look at a diet break is like a weeklong refeed day. If you look at it like *I am going to go crazy and binge on peanut butter and pizza all week*, you will be killing your progress. Look at it this way: a diet break is like a week where you get to have more freedom, higher macros, a break from the feeling of starvation, a break from the feeling of low macros, low leptin, and who knows - your sex hormones may even come back up a little.

IIFYM is affiliated to diet breaks like a big company is affiliated with a lot of smaller companies, like a product is affiliated with a marketplace, like an Internet marketer is affiliated with a cheap product. P.S I am a bit of an Internet marketer myself, so if you are an Internet marketer as well, don't take my analogies personal.

When you're counting macros, diet breaks just work much better than they would with someone on a more intuitive approach and definitely better than when on a meal plan.

Let's say your macros are 65F, 325C, 165P, all you need to do is up them a little for your diet break. If you want to be conservative and not gain any body fat and just fill out, let's put you up to

65F, 400C, 165P. If you are looking to have a little more freedom and aren't scared to gain a pound of body fat, go for 70F, 450C, 155P.

Try this with a meal plan and you will notice that you have no option to fall back on. If you break out of your meal plan, it's a free for all and free for all's are not good when leptin is low. Going off of a meal plan when leptin is low is like going to the grocery store when you're hungry only 100x worse. Intuitive isn't too much better when it comes to diet breaks.

With an intuitive approach, it would be up to you to not binge eat. You will have no numbers to follow, just that you can eat a little more than you have been dieting on. Whether or not you will binge eat on a diet break from an intuitive approach is predicated completely on how you're wired; it's kind of like standing really close to a fire, you may or may not burn yourself.

Diet breaks on a meal plan are like jumping in a fire, you are going to get burnt, it's up to you as to how badly you get burned. It's easy to burn your whole house down when diet breaking from a meal plan.

- I have already over-covered this so I will not beat you to death by saying flexible dieting is an education, but just in case you're thinking about disregarding that fact, IIFYM is an education. It teaches you how to eat more mindfully because you learn just how much fat, carb, and protein was actually in that little 6-inch sub, and how much fat was in the little egg and cheese Mc-fatass thing you just ate.

- You start to understand that losing and gaining weight is actually simple - macros in vs. macros out, or calories burned from energy expenditure vs. calories consumed in food. Even if you don't choose IIFYM as your soul method, I believe everyone should learn IIFYM just for its educational values.

- Because I know so much about macros, and what it takes to get my body into shape, I don't even have to count macros to get to 10% body fat. Eating really lean requires me to be much more precise, so I count macros to get shredded, but not year-round. I have years of experience counting macros, I have done meal plans, intuitive eating, and an assortment of fad diets, but IIFYM was the only eating protocol to allow me to reach sub 8% body fat.

- As far as getting shredded, in my opinion, counting macros is the best way to go. 95% of people won't get shredded using an intuitive approach, and meal plans leave you with cravings because you're very restricted on what you can eat.

   Being restrictive on food choices attributes largely to post diet binging. I am not personally a huge fan of diet plans for contest prep, maybe photo shoots, but not contest prep. When counting macros, you're very accurate, and you have the added benefit of diversity. There is no other form of dieting that allows you to be highly accurate while still allowing you to have an occasional pre workout doughnut.

There are two things that can throw off a diet that is meant to get you shredded. The first thing is a diet that constricts you to eating only a few different foods when you're habitually used to eating a much higher variety of foods. If you are dieting to get shredded, and restricted to only a couple of food choices, it can be very draining. You can't go out to eat with your friends, you can't eat at family events, you can't have the occasional fun meal, you can't have a beer or a glass of wine, etc.

For a select few, this is ok, but for the majority, this is bad. You will sneak and cheat, because you're eating habits permit you to eat just a little bit of cereal, or just one cookie. Then, you're done. You may be making progress but the habitual want for diversity in your diet overpowers the want to get shredded.

Now, not only have you given up on your meal plan, but you now have the idea that you can't get shredded; you're the exception, others can do it just not you. It's not that you can't - it's just that you're following the wrong dieting protocol for your personally. Meal plans aren't for everyone. You will need to regain a healthy relationship with food and then opt for the flexible dieting approach on the next go around, and I can almost promise you that it will work much better for you, just as long as you put in the work.

The second thing that could keep you from

getting lean is inconsistency. What I am saying is that intuitive eating will not work for 99% of people looking to get into contest shape. It may work to get you relatively lean, but not shredded.

Intuitive eating is great, but the margin of error in a diet that is not being weighed out nor macronutrient counted, is severe. It is possible to think you are on a deficit of 200-300 calories, but because you are only eyeballing your foods, you are actually at caloric maintenance or even on a surplus of 50.

When you're really bulked up at 14+ percent body fat or more, the intuitive approach works great just to get you back down to a lean 10-12% body fat. But getting stage lean, 5-7% body fat, requires profound accuracy. There must be little to no margin of error when getting shredded; getting shredded is an art.

The diet, the training and the mindset require the focus of an artist and the consistency, devotion, dedication and determination of a one percenter. Getting shredded for stage is the phenomenon where artistry meets athleticism. As such, the diet must be up to par. The only two dieting protocols that can be used to get one shredded and stage ready are either a **Diet Plan** or **Counting Macros, i.e.** flexible dieting.

- There are no time restrictions on IIFYM. You can eat 8 meals a day with equal portions or follow intermittent fasting. In most diet protocols you have to eat 5-6 meals a day with equal portion sizes and have the meals every 2 and a half to 3 hours. With flexible dieting, you fit your macros around your schedule, not your schedule around your meal plan. You don't have to eat equal portions of fat, carb, and protein in every meal, do as you please, just hit your macros by the end of the day.

I actually recommend eating mainly protein throughout the day and save as many fat and carbs as possible so that you can have a nice satisfying dinner. This is of course for people who are cutting. When bulking, you will have more fats and carbs to play around with, so saving macros for later will be a little less important. Flexible dieting allows you to be "flexible" with food timing, food amounts, food types, and eating frequency.

IIFYM Conclusion

Now that I've given you all of the info on flexible dieting, is it for you? That is a question only you can answer. IIFYM works well for a lot of people but it does have its downfalls. I am not glorifying or knocking on IIFYM, I am giving you the correct context to see IIFYM for what it really is. If you are really into learning about food, your body and the macronutrients, and you want to compete in any sort of physique competition at any time in the future, it's a great idea to learn flexible dieting whether you marry it or not.

Don't get me wrong; flexible dieting is not the be all, end all. For those who are highly overweight and need to lose 100+ pounds, intuitive eating may be more attractive as a long term eating protocol. If you are a fitness athlete in a long term bulking stage, I believe intuitive dieting is the way to go.

The thing is, I have seen people lose 100 pounds on flexible dieting and bodybuilders use IIFYM habitually all year-round. I am giving you the keys; which door you open is completely your decision. There are several different macro counting apps that make counting macros seamless, MyFitnessPal is the favorite of mine and many others, which is why I am providing you with an entire subchapter called MyFitnessPal Hacks, later on in the book.

INTUITIVE EATING (I.E.)

What is intuitive eating? Intuitive eating is the other cool diet that is fighting for our hearts; it's an IIFYM vs. Intuitive Eating warzone out here. Neither really have a heads up but both approaches have some really powerful benefits, as well as downfalls. Intuitive style is more of a free spirited type of diet, whereas IIFYM is structured by numbers.

Let me start this off by saying that my lifestyle is a cross between IIFYM and intuitive. Most of the time I do ok with intuitive, but when I need accuracy on my side, I lean back towards IIFYM. Ok, let's get into what intuitive is.

Intuitive Eating?

Intuitive is a way of eating that teaches you how to have a healthy relationship with food. Intuitive was created to help people have a healthy relationship with food, so they become an expert of their own body. To learn intuitive eating means to learn the difference between physical and emotional feelings and to gain a sense of body wisdom.

Think of it as a process of making peace with food, letting go, and detaching from any bad or unhealthy relationships with food. This way you won't be sitting and thinking about your next meal distracted from reality. This style of dieting/eating is based off learning to respond to your inner body cues. We were all born with the mental wiring to eat intuitively.

The issue is, our nature is greatly affected by our environment. In some cases, our habitual eating habits are completely dependent on our childhood experiences. Some of us have tied in eating with emotions and feelings, i.e. we use food as a drug, as an escapism. Some of us overeat habitually, which leads us to look a certain way and feel a certain way. Some of us undereat habitually, which leads us to believe that we will always be small, that it will always be hard to grow.

Most of us are brought up burdened with certain beliefs, some of them self-fabricated, some of them were told to us by dickheads, and some of them were marketed to us in order to persuade us to buy a product that would give us the after result we wanted. You would be pleasantly surprised to learn how much of your beliefs on dieting, food, and your body are completely false. Your inner wisdom to be eating for your own satiety levels seems simple right?

The problem is this so called "inner wisdom" is covered with myths and lies about food, dieting and your own expectations of your body and what's possible. The basis of intuitive is simply this: eat until you are about 80-90% full, which should be common sense. While it may be common sense, we are already primed to eat a certain way, following strict meal timing, food restrictions, making sure to always finish your food, etc. These things may have hurt you in the long run much more than they helped you in the short term.

Eating Disorder Madness

If you are into bodybuilding or are just a fellow fitness enthusiast, you may know the effects that dieting can have on your relationship with food. In some cases, meal plans that are highly restrictive, along with just being on a caloric deficit for a long period of time, can actually create eating disorders.

I don't think it's healthy for 90% of people to believe they must eat every 3 hours. I don't believe it's healthy to think you have to eat breakfast, or that if you eat after 8pm at night you'll gain fat. Those beliefs can absolutely kill your relationship to food and prime you for eating disorders.

Want to hear something funny? I am a competitive natural bodybuilder as well as a powerlifter; I don't eat breakfast, only a coffee and 2 tbsp. of coconut oil. I only eat 3 meals a day, and no they aren't timed. My dinner is my largest meal; I eat like a king and then pass out. I maintain a lean physique year-round.

There are tons of myths that we believe; some of them we even live by. We are living on mythical ideologies! We all have certain eating behaviors that either keep us fat or keep us super skinny, it doesn't matter which end of the spectrum you fall on, intuitive eating helps free you from all of the bullshit that is holding you back from looking and feeling the way you want to. Personally, I have been on both sides, I have habitually overeaten the wrong foods and been suicidal, and I've also been mind-fucked by being on a caloric deficit for a year to the point where I was hardly eating because I was addicted to seeing the scale drop, even though I was burning my own hard earned muscle to dust by doing so.

Bad relationships with food are widely underestimated. Even for people who aren't looking to build a physique, bad relationships with food will ruin your life. Eating Cheetos mindlessly while playing Call of Duty and drinking Mountain Dew will leave you fat and unhappy. Ask me how I know this...

Eating no carbs at all because someone told you that the way to get shredded was to eat zero carbs, will make you want to kill your friends and family when they do anything that frustrates you in your volatile low carb state.

You will also build a long list of cookies, doughnuts, pizza, and Chinese buffet items that you will eat once the low carb diet ends. Then you binge all the way past your starting bodyweight and possibly even further. In mere weeks you gain back the weight that took you several months to lose. It will take several more months to think about food like a normal human being again. The cravings us bodybuilders have for peanut butter is just abnormal, you may be able to relate to this. When you go completely against your nature and eat because of culture, obligation or emotion, it usually ends badly for yours truly.

Forget About Short Term Diets

Forget about the next fad diet in the article in the magazine tray in your bathroom. Forget about the weight loss pills that promise you to lose 30 pounds in a month. If you're a skinny person, forget about the high calorie mass gainer diet that packs on 10 pounds of muscle in two weeks. "GET FUCKING MAD AT THESE BLATENT LIES." Get mad that marketers are marketing something to everyone that will not benefit them in the long-term, in the big picture.

Stop thinking there is some magnificent diet or way

of eating that is going to get you shredded and jacked in a matter of weeks, even months. Stop bouncing from program to program thinking this diet will get you better results than the last one.

Want to know a secret? Most of the diets being marketed to you by IFBB pro bodybuilders and Hollywood personalities, are highly fictional. These people don't eat like this all of the time, only for a few months to get into shape to take that picture. To top that off, many magazine covers are highly molested by Photoshop in order to deliver the perfect image, the perfect perception. You, the customers, need to see the perfect image of the perfect physique at this precise moment in the book store; that way you will hold this perception in your head until you go and buy the supplement, jump on the pumped up meal plan, go buy the program, go buy the fat melting sweat belt, or purchase the muscle building, electrical muscle pulsation thing.

Stop thinking this way and start thinking long-term. Don't think "diet," don't think 30-day, don't think short term numbers or results at all. Think lifestyle, think relationship to food.

Eat When Hungry

Eat when you're hungry and don't think you need to eat certain foods or that other foods are absolutely evil. Eat mindfully; don't go stuff your face at the speed of light with simple sugars and short chain fats, but at the same time don't blame that one doughnut on the obesity epidemic of America.

It's not that little doughnut's fault, it's our conditioning as a culture, or beliefs, or habitual overeating problems.

Some of us are really overweight and some of us can't gain weight. Both are problems of the mind - mindless habits that lead us into a lifestyle that contradicts how we want to look and feel.

Eating to Lose Body Fat

You have been primed to always finish your food because the starving kids in Africa will be angry with you if you leave any food uneaten. If this is the case, they are also angry with you for not helping them not be starving, but this is beside the point.

If you are starting to get full, put a sheet of saranwrap over your food and eat it later. You have this whole "all or nothing" eating delusion in your head, don't you? You're either going to starve yourself eating spinach, lettuce and a few craisins, or binge eat on Japanese carryout and later some Ben & Jerry's.

This whole extreme thing is killing you, nobody actually wins this way. You think all of the people that look good starved themselves on spinach, lettuce and an almond to get into great shape? No, nobody does that, nothing lasting ever comes from anything quick and extreme. Start out by simply being mindful of your bipolar eating philosophy.

Then act to get rid of this toxic eating mindset. Eat until you're 80-90% full, eat mostly foods that are highly nutritious and not calorie dense. Look back to part one of the book for a list of carb, fat, and protein sources that will help you be more full and energetic.

If you want that doughnut, eat one, but realize that eating the whole box and then telling yourself that tomorrow you will eat leaves all day isn't going to get you anything but diabetes. Get the idea out of your head that there are these perfectly healthy people out there. Even people who are in amazing shape eat what they want when they want it.

That is one of the biggest reasons that they can maintain a healthy, lean physique. When you tell yourself you can't have a food, it's bad, it is evil that will do nothing more than develop an intense craving for the food until you binge on it.

Once you have given in to your innermost intense cravings you will be binging on that food with candle's lit, your favorite song playing, and fireworks going off in your head. That is not healthy, you fabricated the development all by yourself from the extreme deprivation of that food that you wanted so badly. Once you finish binging and you go into a food coma and need a blanket to cover your food baby, and are drowning in your own tears of self-hate, you will realize how much this sucks.

Food isn't a drug by nature, but you can transform anything in your head into a drug if you're not careful. This is another issue that overweight and obese people deal with, they have an assortment of carefully developed food drugs.

This is the reason that I said IIFYM is not a good idea for people who already have food addictions. IIFYM forces you to think about food because you are having to calculate food and hit your macros. If you have a junk food addiction, this will most likely support that addiction because you will just fill your macros with these foods.

Anyone with a bad relationship with food needs to start out with intuitive eating as their form of dieting or way of eating until they get a handle on their relationship with food. Your relationship will 100% dictate your health and your physique, so this must be a priority over weight loss or weight gain.

Your relationship to food is the foundation under your house; if the foundation is weak, the house will fall apart every time. Intuitive eating is the foundation that is missing with all people who have terrible relationships with food.

Eating to Grow on Intuitive

If you're underweight and seem to stay underweight, the simple way to put it is that you're not putting enough calories into your body to create a caloric surplus. You most likely eat constantly and tell everyone that you eat a lot of food. You eat all day but can't gain any weight.

You don't need a bunch of mass gainer shakes or steroids, you just need to stop snacking on skittles and potato chips and actually eat some food. You my friend have been gifted with a fast metabolism and high levels of leptin. You may not see it as a gift now but you will have a much easier time than 90% of fitness athletes when it comes to getting in shredded shape for photo shoots or in contest shape.

Eating intuitively to grow simply means eating more foods that will actually give you some energy, some bang for your buck. You have the opposite problem of an overweight person, where the overweight person is addicted to food, you practically forget to eat, or didn't realize that you only ate 2,000 calories today and it was from candy and junk food.

Do you really want to grow? If you want to build some muscle and not be skinny forever, you need to retrain your brain. When you get little hunger cravings, what do you go for? Maybe a bag of chips? Possibly just whatever random food item you can find, or maybe just a soda?

This needs to change if you want to build some muscle. You need to be eating like a man. Chicken, steak, beef, fish, eggs and poultry for protein. For carbs: oats, rice, pastas, potatoes, fruit and veggies. Add in some fat sources like coconut oil, almonds, assorted nuts, flaxseed oil and cold pressed, unrefined olive oil. Relate back to the first section of the book to find an assortment of fat, carb and protein sources to go for.

The great thing in your case, is that after you have changed your habitual eating habits to real, unprocessed, nutrient dense foods, this is where you can add back in the fun foods. Ice cream is a great mass gainer, yogurt is great, enjoy yourself. The thing is, your metabolism may be too fast to just gain weight from nutrition dense whole foods, but you also won't get anywhere living off of junk food.

When you are eating a diet based on whole food, and you add in the fun stuff on top of that, then you can expect to finally start to grow! After a while, eating more and eating better will come natural, it will become intuitive. You have to make the correlation in your brain that doing x every day equal x results. Once you subconsciously correlate eating more and eating better to making "GAINZ," eating big will become a part of you.

Cast Out the Monsters in Your Head

If you have good and evil voices in your head, then I am talking directly to you. Don't worry, this happens to a lot of people, and it's not that hard to get rid of. You know the voice that pops up when you haven't eaten very much all day and says, "good job you may be less of a fat ass tomorrow." The voice then says, "you can't eat that or you're a terrible person." The voice then says "yes, just one slice of pie," then 10 minutes later you're very angry with that lying, cheating asshole in your head.

We all have these voices; we need to forget about them. Here is the thing my friend, you created these food angels and demons so you can erase them. Why did you create them? You believed having some sort of food morals, rewards and punishment would help you somehow. I know, I know you didn't purposely set out to do this, nobody does.

Don't blame yourself and stop shaming yourself. You're not wrong for wanting a slice of pizza, you shouldn't have to sneak around in your head and be private about eating a slice of birthday cake.

You have accidentally created this whole judiciary law system in your head. You must not cheat, you must not eat from this list of evil foods, you must eat over x calories, you must stay strict 24/7. You are like a sneaky criminal in your own subconscious; you feel like you don't even deserve a lot of things because subconsciously, you have degraded the hell out of your self-confidence and ability to follow through with things.

Here is the thing: the drug addict in your head was created in your head, justified by fictional insecurities and false boundaries. You may have destroyed your relationship to food, and your self-love in the process, now it's time to get it all back.

When you don't eat a whole lot on one day because you were busy or just not hungry, think nothing of it, it just was. No rewards, no "that's how I need to be all the time." If you want a slice of pizza one day, a slice of cake one day, a bowl of ice-cream, just give yourself what you want. It's not a crime, you're not cheating, you are not going against your morals, you're not a fat ass, you are "YOU."

If you don't have these morals, these self-restrictions, these laws, then you won't feel like you are under pressure or doing something wrong. You won't obsess over what you're eating, and what you absolutely can't eat. There are no bad foods, there are whole nutrient dense foods, and processed less nutrient dense foods.

Eat mostly whole, healthy food, eat until you're 80-90% full, and don't feel obligated to finish your food. Don't challenge the voices in your head, forget they ever existed. Trying to get away from something forces it to become more apparent in your life. The only way to get away from the voices in your head is to acknowledge that they are indeed real, and then let them go, you don't need them anymore.

Eat What You Want When You Want

Don't constrict yourself to any kind of meal timing, meal frequency or times you must eat or must not eat. Eat when it comes natural. Doing this will keep you from being food focused.

Eating in a way that is the easiest and least stressful for you will make your eating experience much more rewarding. You will find that putting your eating into your life instead of putting your life into your eating is highly rewarding and leaves you feeling fuller after each meal. When you tell yourself I must eat breakfast, breakfast is the most important meal of the day, it does nothing really good for your relationship with food.

Here is a shocker, it doesn't matter: breakfast isn't the most important meal of the day, and it's just a meal. Not eating after a certain time is also pointless and has no merit, ooh, and eating more frequently doesn't do anything spectacular for your metabolism. I will be sure to nail these facts into your head.

There are studies showing all of those things do affect metabolism, fat loss and fat gain, but they're all thrown way out of context; context is everything in the health and fitness space. Mentally, the more you change your eating frequency, timing, types of food, and eating environments, the more you will feel like you are on a diet. We want to mitigate this feeling of you being on a diet because intuitive eating isn't a diet, it's a lifestyle change.

I may call intuitive eating a "diet" or "eating protocol," but I only do so to put the correct context on intuitive as being one of the 3 types of eating protocols. The goal of intuitive eating is simply to build a relationship with food that is so strong that it doesn't require your constant attention; you need not actively think about food until you are actually eating it. That is the way it was meant to be in nature, but somewhere along the line we decided to take nature into our own hands.

There is always all this talk about what is efficient, what is scientifically proven to do X, Y, and Z. I say fuck that, do what is natural, do what makes you happy. If a way of eating or a certain diet makes you sad, or you're ready to get it over with, then you need to find one that you can live with long-term, one that isn't hard to live with.

You are probably the type of person that has issues with every other type of diet other than intuitive, if you hate any and every diet you have ever been on. You are tired of thinking about food timing, so don't, don't even think about timing and frequency anymore. Just eat a diet rich in nutrient dense carbs and fat, and lean proteins. If you want something tasty, eat it whenever it pops in your head.

This whole eating thing isn't as hard or stressful as you may have made it out to be in your head. You just like to make things over complicated, but not today my friend.

Stop Eating your Feelings

Whatever is stressing you out, making you feel uneasy, whatever you're worried about, you can't eat it away, so stop trying to. There is anxiety, loneliness, boredom, and even anger and sadness.

When you are faced with these emotions, realize them, and don't mindlessly binge to drown them out. This is only going to make you feel worse. When you feel sadness or anxiety creeping up on you, realize it and face it.

We all get sad, it's natural to be sad from time to time. We all get anxiety at times, life can be stressful. Sometimes out of our anger comes sadness and vice versa.

My suggestion to you when this happens is this: go read a book, listen to an audio book, do something uplifting and mentally strengthening, go to the book store and get a small coffee and read about something that interests you, go to the movies, just you, a movie and a coke zero. If you are going to the gym every day, or at least 3 to 4 days per week, focus on getting a great workout, or go on a walk or a run.

If you're bored, seriously, get off your ass and do something. No, eating doesn't count, because then you will be sad. Find something to fill your time with that will amount to something, a better you, a stronger you, a smarter you, a more creative you.

Life is about building a reality that you are proud of. If you are bored, then you are wasting your own time not having fun or being productive, which is also fun if you're being productive doing something you're passionate about. Eating because your bored is something most of us have done but there is any easy fix - stop being bored.

We all feel lonely from time to time, but we don't have to. If you're not bored, then you won't be lonely. A bit of advice - become habitually un-bored before you go searching for a soul mate.

This feeling of loneliness is just a feeling of you having nothing to put your passion into, you just need to find something to create, something to make yours. Start the business you have always wanted to start, apply for that job you want deep down, study and train for that lifestyle you want to live.

Food will be the last thing on your mind if you are happy and busy. You need to be busy before you even worry about the lonely problem. If you're busy, and you just have a couple of friends, you won't be lonely; no need to even worry about that part of your life.

Food doesn't have to be your coping mechanism. You don't need one, you need to get out of the state you're in, just do it, change your own life. The relationship with food is a big part of that change.

Stop Starving Your Feelings

Plot twist? Yep, I know about you guys, too. You underweight and adrenally tapped. You use a lot of caffeine, a lot of stimulants and get little sleep. You stress about tomorrow and wish you had a better yesterday.

With all of these stress hormones and neurological stimulants, you're in fight or flight mode all the time. You my friend have the ability to think yourself into a dark hole that subsequently leads you to starvation. You have come to welcome these feelings or at least you think it's a normal thing that's ok.

It's not ok. It may seem ok right now, but eventually you will run into health problems. Running on E all of the time will keep your body in fight for flight mode. If you're a guy, your testosterone levels will start to drop, along with many other important hormones.

If you are a girl, your estrogen levels will drop, as well as other valuable hormones. Your hormones won't be the only thing that's affected; you will also affect your muscles, joints, ligaments and mental wellbeing. If your brain isn't getting glucose or ketones, there won't be any production of happy hormones like serotonin.

Contrary to popular belief, depression, anxiety, bipolar, sadness, homesickness, any many other "disorders" for most people aren't actually disorders, they're reactions to circumstances. Depression can usually be cured by simply eating better and becoming more physical, working out. I prescribe this for just about every single so called "mental illness" out there.

Eating highly nutritious carbs, having the proper nitrogen balance in the body by eating enough protein, and having the proper brain function by eating the necessary fats, puts you in an environment to produce the hormones you need to be happy.

Working out also does this. It's perfectly normal to go through things in life and stress out, freak out, cry, be sad. We all go through breakups, deaths, loss of passion, failures, pain, feeling lost, feeling stabbed in the back. You need to make sure you're eating during these times. You probably won't be able to eat 100% normally, but make sure you're eating something.

You want to build muscle? You want to become stronger, more powerful, healthy, a better you? You need to keep feeding your mind and body even when you don't feel like it. If you have already become familiar with the feeling of anxiety in the body, and disregarded eating because you didn't want to eat, it's time right now to refeed your mind and body. Tell yourself I need to eat to grow, to eat to be strong, to eat to have a healthy metabolism.

You're not going to build any muscle, get shredded, or be sexy when starving yourself, you will just be skinny and unhealthy. You can't starve your feelings away, you just can't, so EAT! When you get hungry and then you think about something that stresses you out, find a way to eat something even if it's a small protein shake and some fruit, just eat something.

By doing this, you are establishing that you have control over how thoughts effect you. Do this consistently and eventually the thoughts will become less and less, and eating when you're hungry will become intuitive despite your anxiety.

Face your emotions but realize that you can still eat. You can still live life when faced with adversities, when faced with heartache and mental agony.

Accept Your Genetics

Everyone is born a certain way with their own genetic blueprint. Some people will never be able to maintain sub 10% body fat levels year-round without feeling like shit, while others will have a hard time ever bulking out of 10% body fat.

Some people genetically pull a lot of weight on deadlift, and some people genetically bench-press a lot of weight, even if they stop working out for months. Some people can eat 5,000 calories and be shredded, other people will get fat going over 2,500.

If your metabolism is high, you may call yourself a hard gainer. If it's easier for you to gain weight, you may call yourself an endomorph. Instead of labeling one's self, what I like to do is say, fuck it, this is my body, my metabolism, I am going to create something out of it. Either side can complain about what type of metabolism they have.

Here is the thing: everyone has certain genetic gifts, yes everyone, yes even you. When you are blessed with a fast metabolism, you will be able to eat more than anyone else without gaining too much body fat. If you are the type where it's easier for you to gain weight, you will have a much easier time gaining muscle than the person with the sonic metabolism.

Some people genetically are taller, which gives them the ability to have a better stride than the shorter person, and because they are a bigger person, when they build muscle they will be much larger looking. Some people are genetically shorter, and won't have as great of a stride; however, because their limbs are shorter, the bar has a shorter path to travel to hit depth on bench-press, squat, and deadlift.

Therefore, the shorter person will have an easier time building strength pound for pound and will have an easier time building a more dense-looking physique. One thing stands true: once you understand your own genetics, your gifts, your weaknesses, you can eat intuitively to be the best "YOU" possible.

When you learn to accept your genetics and create a plan that will complement them, which includes eating for your specific goals, you will see tremendous changes in the body. You will become the most powerful, complete version of yourself. Don't argue with your genetics; if gaining weight is easy for you, stop eating when you begin to feel full. If gaining weight is impossible, eat more, eat more, eat more. Eat for your genetics and goals - it will become as easy as practicing something consistently and will make it intuitive.

Eat for Health & Enjoy Your Food

Contrary to popular belief, healthy food tastes good. I don't know where the idea that "if it's healthy, it won't taste good" came from, but it's simply false. Eat the foods that you enjoy while giving your body what it needs, i.e. vitamins, minerals, fiber, and high quality sources of fat, carb and proteins.

It's extremely satisfying to eat something that tastes amazing and also helps lead you towards your goals, whether fat loss or muscle gain. It's not about perfection, it's about consistency. Eating one snack that you're craving isn't going to suddenly make you gain weight. Enjoying yourself one night won't create a nutrient deficiency.

Just like flexible dieting, with intuitive the goal is always to eat mostly nutrient dense and filling foods, and fitting in the foods that you crave when the craving comes about.

Use Intuitive Eating for What It Is

Intuitive eating was meant to make you happy, to create a relationship with food that allows you to stay healthy on auto pilot. Intuitive is the only form of eating that allows you to eat towards your fat loss or muscle gain goals without counting numbers, without creating a structured meal plan, and without having to really have food as thought.

You shouldn't be thinking about food all day, 24 hours a day, 7 days a week, 12 months a year. We were naturally meant to eat for our bodies. Eating was meant to be an experience, it was meant to be enjoyable. We are meant to eat until lightly full. We aren't bears, so we don't hibernate, which means we aren't meant to eat until we are about to faint and store tons of body fat.

We are also not meant to be stressed all of the time and never eat because we always feel sick. Simply learn how to eat when hungry because of hunger, not because of emotion, not because of boredom, not because it's been 3 hours and you need to eat again, but eat when hungry. It's a game changing idea! We can actually just eat when hungry and it will solve a lot of our problems? Yep, it's true, it's just not that simple, which you now know.

Intuitive Eating Cons

- If you are someone who likes structure, any structure at all, then intuitive is not for you. There is no structure whatsoever in intuitive eating. No counting fat, carb, protein, no calories to hit, no meal plan, no eating boundaries.

It's up to you to eat the right food and eat a diet that is highly nutritious with complex carbs, fruits and veggies, omega fatty acids, MCT's, and high quality proteins. Some people need structure or they will be completely lost.

If you are the type of person that at the end of the day needs some sort of destination to hit in terms of your eating protocol, then intuitive is not for you. When following intuitive you will be looking for hunger ques, putting yourself in enjoyable eating environments and eating until 80-90% full.

If you are someone that is completely out of tune with your body's hunger signs or full signs, maybe you need a little bit of structure until you can better understand your body. If you are you someone who isn't looking for all out IIFYM or meal plans but needs a little structure, then I recommend mixing two styles of eating.

Come up with a fat, carb, and protein target to hit for the day, for example 65 fat, 300 carb, 160 protein. Don't break your neck to count these macros, give yourself a roundabout target so for fats your goal would be anywhere from 50-70 grams, your carbs anywhere from 300 to 350, for protein 150-170 grams a day.

Now, these macros aren't for the sake of really using macros as a practice, but serve as a slight backbone to your intuitive approach until you are ready for 100% intuitive eating. You can also mix intuitive with a meal plan, have your meals slightly structured out, but don't be obligated to finish them, just eat until full.

If you want to swap out one meal for another, or completely change a meal, go for it. If you want to have some one thing out of the blue that you are craving, go for it.

Whether mixing intuitive with a diet plan or IIFYM, just remember you're still looking to improve your hunger signals, relationship to food and eating environment. Never feel obligated to eat a certain amount of meals; finish an entire meal at one sitting if full before it's finished, or be restrictive.

You may never want to go completely intuitive, and that's fine, structure is great, just make sure that you lead a healthy relationship with food no matter which form or forms of dieting you follow.

- Intuitive is a lot like IIFYM in one way - you will make of it what you will make of it, I think you know where I am going with this. The form of dieting you go with, the form of eating structure that works best for you, depends highly on your psychology.

You could take advantage of the "eat what you want" part of intuitive and prance around saying that you're on intuitive eating, but you're actually intuitively eating shit. Intuitive, like IIFYM, is designed so that your daily diet is based off of primarily nutrient dense foods.

On both eating protocols you can fit in the things you crave when you get the cravings.

According to intuitive, you should eat the foods you crave whenever you crave them. But what if you already do that? Hmmm, now we have reached a grey area in intuitive. What if you already have a great relationship with food, but it's a great relationship with highly unhealthy and calorie dense, processed food?

Just like that great relationship you think you have with that asshole you're dating or married to, it's time to cut it. You don't need intuitive or IIFYM, you need to wake up and look at what you're doing to yourself.

Your entire diet needs an overhaul, and then once you have gotten rid of what needs to be cast out, then you can think about intuitive or IIFYM. Luckily, you have this whole book, so you can learn what to eat, start eating it, and then rebuild your relationship with food around food that contributes to your life, and not food that destroys it.

You need to put on your training wheels, before you can become a bike you have to be a tricycle, before you can fly you have to crawl, before you can be healthy you have to get rid of the filth. That entire pizza you eat on the weekends, that huge bowl of pasta you eat for dinner, that container of ice-cream you eat to snack on, that shit has to stop.

This goes for highly overweight people who can't lose any weight, and underweight people. If you're highly underweight, learn to eat actual food, not little baby snacks of chips and candy. First, you have to see the problem and get completely rid of it; you need to be administered the right form of eating for yourself at this current point in time.

If it's a complete eating overhaul that you need, whether you're super skinny or highly overweight you need to tread lightly and be careful with intuitive. You need to change what you eat and then start to structure it. You may be better starting out on a personalized meal plan that can be mixed with intuitive when ready.

What's a personalized meal plan you may ask? This is a meal plan that's personalized to give you all of the foods you're not currently eating that your body needs for proper function. At the end of the day, it's up to you to decide what direction best suits you. If you don't know, this is where online coaching can be valuable to you. Sometimes you may not know what is best for you; a little help may give you the confidence you need to better understand your mind and body for years to come.

It's sad, but most people will never understand the forms of dieting, when to start, what to eat, what they may be doing wrong, etc. because they never take the time to find out. They don't even care about their health or physique enough to commit $100 a month to someone who can help change their life. You're not silly for trying to understand your mind and body and how they work together, you're ten steps ahead of the people who don't care.

- Intuitive eating is not very precise, which takes it out of the game when it comes to getting shredded. When you're dieting to get really lean and shredded, accuracy is key, accuracy and consistency. Intuitive is not very accurate at all as compared to IIFYM or meal plans.

It is possible to get relatively lean on intuitive, but when it comes to getting shredded for contest prep, I just don't think it's going to cut it. The fact that you're not really tracking numbers, not weighing food, not really creating any structure, makes this a terrible eating protocol decision for contest preppers. You may think you're eating 30-40 carbs with that potato, but if you have never had experience weighing food and counting macros, your potato may in fact be 60 carbs.

You may think that you just ate 6 ounces of chicken but in fact you ate 8.5 ounces, and you did this for 3 meals. You may think that little bit of cheesecake isn't that bad, but it actually has 30 grams of fat and 75 carbs. Boom, you're eating almost 1,000 calories more than you realize.

You're either going to be maintaining your weight or putting yourself on a slight caloric surplus; congratulations, you're on what we call a "lean bulk" even though you think you're on a cut.

• If you don't have a background in meal plans or IIFYM, you may have no context for intuitive eating. How can an intuitive eating plan work when you don't know exactly how much fat, carb, and protein are in your food choices?

If you have never weighed a bowl of cereal, never weighed a potato, never weighed chicken, never weighed rice, never weighed your fruit, never weighed your ice-cream, how will you have eyeball to macro context? You won't. If you don't have eyeball context on food, you may be 1,000 calories over what you think you are eating, or 1,000 calories under what you think you are eating.

In theory, eating until you're 80-90% full should work for everyone. The problem is some of us are just so wired to eat until we are in a coma, or bored of the food we are eating, that we have no context on how full we are, we have only *eat this, eat that, should I stop now?*

Nope, I believe I will have some cereal, then some ice-cream, now I need something salty, aha potato chips! You have no idea what universe 80% full exists in, you need to get on a diet plan and weigh some damn food. You need to learn about macros for the sake of understanding that eating is not a free for all. Yes, you want to have a healthy relationship with food but you need to understand food before you can have any sort of relationship with it.

Most of us don't just wake up having context in regards to macronutrients, micronutrients, how much of each we need to reach our goals, and how much our dog needs to reach his goals. I started out using meal plans; for 4 years a meal plan was my go to eating protocol. Meal plans taught me about what foods I needed to prioritize in my diet to make gains, to stay lean, to perform in the gym.

I learned about the importance of protein on a bulk and on a cut, that I needed to eat mainly complex carbs and green veggies for health and performance, and also that I needed to get good sources of fat in my diet as well.

At around 18 years of age I began counting macros, which took my understanding of food and my body to another level. I started to understand how much protein was in 6, 8, 10, and 12 ounces of chicken, fish, and steak, and also what that looked like from an eyeball prospective. I learned the importance of saving macros for later on in the day so that I could enjoy being normal with my friends; I learned how to budget and time my macros to create an enjoyable eating environment while staying lean year-round.

I also learned the difference between a 100-gram and 200-gram apple, I learned what 40 grams of oatmeal looks like, what 100 grams of ice-cream looks like, etc. Counting macros taught me more about my body and food than any education could have. I learned what amount of food I needed to eat at certain bodyweights to lose or gain weight.

I also learned that my fat as a macro has a big effect on weight loss for me. Some people do better with lower carbs and higher fat; personally I do better on lower fat, higher carbs. I have counted macros for almost 3 years and now I follow intuitive eating most of the year and switch back to IIFYM when I am looking to get shredded. The thing is, I would have no context to follow intuitive eating if not for my years of meal plans and IIFYM.

It's not a necessity for everyone to count macros, but it's a free education that beats about anything you can pay for in terms of learning about food and your body. I will say over and over again, get a coach. It's hard to understand how to manipulate macronutrients, or have the context and understanding of when you should drop or raise carbs, as well as fat.

Intuitive eating is much different for an overweight person who needs to lose weight than for an athlete looking for optimal performance and to build a strong and powerful physique. Intuitive wasn't created for performance athletes; so when we are looking at intuitive for athletes, we need to look at your understanding of your body, food, macronutrients, etc.

Intuitive is 100% predicated on context because you can't be intuitive without first understanding the magic behind the intuition. The only reason I am personally able to do so well on intuitive is because I have years of structured dieting in my subconscious, which makes eating to grow intuitive for me, eating to get shredded intuitive for me, hitting my fiber and getting in valuable nutrients intuitive for me. Intuition doesn't just pop up. It first needs maturity in the form of education.

Intuitive Eating Pros

- If you hate structure, intuitive is for you. Are you the type of person that is revolted by counting macros, and can't stand the thought of having your meals planned out every day, for days in advance? You're not alone.

There are a lot of people that don't really enjoy having to count macros or eat according to a meal plan. Intuitive eating won't hold you to certain eating timings; you won't have to stick to only a couple of food choices, and you won't have to count anything. Out of the 3 forms of eating, intuitive is the least time consuming and the least food focused.

With that said, it's completely up to you to make smart food choices, create a satisfying eating environment, and eat towards your goals. When intuitive eating, you want to take lifestyle into account: Am I going out to eat tonight? Do I want to have something full of sugar later? Do I want pizza tonight? Do I want to watch a movie with popcorn and candy tonight?

Just like IIFYM, you do need to make sure that when you are going to be eating a lot of calories at night that you plan for it. I don't suggest that you sacrifice healthy fats and carbs in order to have a pizza, popcorn or candy every night, but once a week is perfectly fine.

Make sure to get your protein in. It's easy to get in carbs using the intuitive approach; however, protein can sometimes slip your mind. Remember, without protein, you will lose muscle on a caloric deficit, and even if you're eating on a caloric surplus you won't gain any muscle without getting in enough protein.

There are many different recommendations for protein intake, it depends on body type and goals. Aim for 1 gram of protein per pound of bodyweight. It's not that big of a deal whether you hit .8 grams per bodyweight and 1.2 the next day, the important thing is that you're getting in a good amount of protein every day.

I recommend eating the majority of your protein early on in the day when planning to have a fun night out involving some tasty food items. Since this is intuitive, you won't actually be counting your protein every day, just make sure that you have a couple meals that are high in protein which will lead you towards hitting your bodyweight in protein every day. Hitting protein becomes intuitive very easily so don't overthink it.

Don't overthink any of this stuff because I know you are the type of person that loves to overthink things, which is why you don't do well with too much structure. You will still want to create a nice social eating environment for yourself, which requires you saving some fat and carbs left over for when you know you will take a big stab at them.

Most days you won't have any movie date planned, so just hit your protein, pay attention to your body's hunger cues and eat until 80-90% full. Personally, what I like to do is eat very light or fast early in the day, eat until about 80% full throughout most of the day, and then for dinner eat until 90% full.

Another thing that is helpful to do is eat a very light yet satisfying breakfast, or just a coffee and a lot of water if you prefer fasting, and then eat super high volume but low calorie throughout the day. What do I mean by this? I mean spinach leaves, chopped tomatoes, broccoli, lettuce, cucumbers, and drinking flavored water or green tea, which can all help keep you feeling full throughout the day.

So, we are looking at meals throughout the day like a chicken salad with 85 grams of spinach or more, add tomatoes, cucumbers and lettuce if you want. Also adding a little bit of fruit to your salad meal helps; blueberries, grapes, strawberries, pineapples. Make sure to be light on the fruit, just a handful.

Also, make sure if you use a sauce or a dressing, to get the fat free or reduced fat version and use it very sparingly. Balsamic vinaigrette, and apple cider vinegar are great salad additives. This meal will have a lot of your nutrients in it and should give you great energy and keep you feeling full throughout the day. Another great meal option is a fish and broccoli meal, or a fish and mixed veggies meal.

Make sure to come up with your own tasty blend of seasonings for the fish, and a little salt on the freshly steamed vegetables will do it. Enjoy these meals, enjoy the simplicity of the salad, and have fun making it, be creative, use different ingredients in your salad whenever it is feeling blah. Just make sure to stay away from HFCS sauces, high fat dressings and adding too much fruit. Also, that other meal could be fun as well; you have several different options for your protein source, it could be salmon, cod, tilapia, or even a lean meat, eggs, protein smoothie, etc.

Then for dinner, enjoy yourself a little! Now

I am not giving you a diet plan, just some tips. I personally do well eating 100% intuitively. You may eat however you like, just make sure the way you're eating is not stressing you out and that it's leading you towards your goals, that's what's important.

If you are losing weight too quickly, simply add in more food. If you want to gain weight, add in more complex carbs and fruit. This isn't complicated, I promise. Intuitive is the easiest, most maintainable form of dieting in my opinion. With that said, it's not a free for all; you do need to have a loose game plan to follow every week that leads you towards your goals.

Creating a game plan to go hand and hand with your intuitive eating is easy. Just play your cards right and you will be moving straight towards your goals without even feeling like you're dieting, all while feeling really good about yourself and the foods you're eating.

• Just like there is no cheating with IIFYM, there is no cheating with intuitive. Cheating becomes irrelevant when you become intuitive. If you want something, and it won't stop you from hitting your goals, eat it.

The more you eat things as you want them, the less likely you will ever be to have cravings for anything, and the stronger relationship you will have with food. Isn't reverse psychology cool? The more you give in to your natural wants, the less you will want for anything.

Intuitive gives you a little bit more freedom

than IIFYM because you're not fitting a food item into your macros, you are simply eating. Dieting culture has taught us to be restrictive, don't eat this, structure that, try to dance around eating this, etc.

This has created a culture of negative energy towards food or a negative eating environment. It's also taken all of the enjoyment out of eating, literally to the point that some people would rather die than participate in what they think "dieting" is. The problem lies in the misperception that the definition of "diet" is to live a dreadful life of eating boring food.

The truth is, "diet" means the way you eat. It means the kinds of food that a person, animal or community eats. Somewhere along the lines as a culture we changed the definition of "diet" to a special way of eating which restricts one's self to either lose weight or be healthier.

Here is a simple fact: even if you're eating super nutrient-dense food all day, if you hate what you're eating and it makes you sad or stressed, you're doing more harm than good. Think of the word diet as simply a way of eating, not a negative way of eating - a diet is a template not a structure.

Intuitive is a blessing to many because it has helped people to realize that they shouldn't be super restrictive, they don't need to be super strategic, and dieting is miserable. Eating better, looking better, having the body/physique we want, feeling energetic and powerful - it's not that god given phenomenon that only the genetically gifted can experience.

We all have the power to be who we want to be, in the kitchen, at the gym and in life, and it's not that complicated. Cheating shouldn't exist when it comes to eating. Cheating is human nature disguised as shameful behavior. I am only talking about food here, cheating on your spouse is wrong, and I do not condone this dickhead behavior.

Building the body you want isn't about being perfect, it's about being consistent. The most powerful law of transformation in health and fitness is the law of compounding. The more results you receive from the work you put in, the more results you will strive to create for yourself.

The better you feel by eating in a healthy and satisfying way, the more intuitive it will become; the more you eat foods you want, when you want them, the less you will think about them. You will realize that over the years, eating intuitively to hit goals and maintaining a certain physique and lifestyle isn't much different than someone who is a habitual overeater of processed high calorie food. What you do habitually and consistently over time will create the "you" that looks you in the mirror every day.

- Intuitive eating is great for bodybuilders and physique competitors in the off season. As someone who has used IIFYM, meal plans and intuitive eating, I can tell you that finding a diet that you can live with year-round is crucial.

- Meal plans year-round are completely unnecessary and for most of us, it would take all of the fun out of life. IIFYM can be utilized year-round, but do you really want to count numbers for all eternity? If you do, more power to you.

- Once you have competed in a competition displaying your physique that you built over the year, and then dieted down to low levels of body fat to reveal the muscle, you need a healthy way of eating to fall back on.

- Some people do need structure the first month or two after a competition, but after that I believe every bodybuilder deserves some time to be normal and enjoy interesting and extravagant foods without tracking the fat, carb, and protein in them.

At the same time, if you're hobby or career is based off of your physique, you can't just have a free for all in the off season. Intuitive provides that perfect middle ground between intense, precise dieting and the American diet. If you have been on meal plans or counted macros as a physique athlete, eating intuitively shouldn't be a problem.

Hypothetically, once you have counted macros long enough, you could become completely intuitive to the point where you know your macros intuitively, aha, wormhole in space time continuum. I live in that wormhole; I use intuitive 90% of the time and it works well for me because my subconscious knows that the macros + my relationship with food isn't too shabby so I also know when to eat what I want and when to chill on the junk food. IIFYIE? Is that a thing? It is now!

Using intuitive eating to return your relationship to food back to normal after getting shredded for a show works wonderfully, but it also works great to get you relatively lean while dieting into a show. When the going gets tough, that's when you can make the switch to IIFYM to diet into the show!

If you're a physique athlete or future physique athlete reading this book, just remember, you may be striving to build something that most people will never regard as possible and that is a powerful thing, but you are still human and you do need to give yourself some freedom or you will burn yourself out. Intuitive eating gives us the freedom that meal plans and IIFYM don't. We are in pursuit of the good life, not perfection.

- Just as IIFYM is an education of the numbers, intuitive is an education of the feelings. With IIFYM, you learn how much fat, carb, and protein to eat every day in order to hit your fat loss or muscle building goals.

You also learn what a certain weight of food contains in terms of macros. You even learn what your macros should be at different bodyweights so that you can maintain, drop from or rise from any bodyweight.

Intuitive educates you in a more artistic way. When you look at the education you receive from IIFYM, it's mathematical and precise. Intuitive uses no numbers or super precise ways of being exact. Intuitive teaches you to rely on your natural hunger signals as opposed to eating because you're bored; intuitive teaches you to eat when you're hungry.

You learn to actually enjoy your food, not just choke it down while focused on something else. If you have 100% awareness that you just ate a nice, satisfying meal, you will be less likely to be hungry for a snack later. Eating tasty food and taking the experience in can be one of the most enjoyable parts of life, yet most of us choose to only give half of our attention to our meal, sometimes even less.

If you don't pay attention to your eating, you will not eat more by nature. Think about this, if you have sex with your partner but at the same time you're wondering if your Facebook status will get a lot of likes and if you should work arms or back tomorrow, you are going to disregard the experience, your relationship with this person will start to fade, disconnect. Your relationship to food is already completely faded because you don't pay any attention to the eating experience. Don't worry, you can rebuild a relationship and appreciation for food again.

You just need to give some of your attention back to eating. This makes I.E. an education in focus. Where is your focus? Maybe you should stop trying to focus on more than one thing at once. Fun fact, we can't actually focus on more than one thing at once, not even a computer can do that.

Even a computer alternates its focus from one

thing to another, but the computer does it so fast that we don't realize that it isn't doing multiple things at once. We are also capable of alternating our attention and focus, but that normally causes very bad things to happen to us humans.

We forget something very important and look like an asshole, we forget to eat, we forget that we just ate, we forget about our mother's birthday, we forget to turn the stove off, we forget to go to sleep at night, we forget to pay attention to the road and go to sleep forever taking another person with us. We aren't meant to be thinking about five other things while eating and watching a TV show, nor are we meant to attempt to do any number of other things seemingly simultaneously.

Learn to focus your attention on your food when eating it, learn to do the same with the rest of your life.

- I.E. is an education of the emotions. Do you realize how often your emotions influence your eating? Some of us try to eat our feelings away, some of us try to starve our feelings. Intuitive eating is to see the influences our emotions have on our eating habits and end them.

We don't need to be trying to blunt our emotions with food, or starve them by not eating, or erase them with drugs. If you want to drop your emotions off somewhere, do it at the gym using your hands, feet and iron.

You learn so much from I.E.; you learn to handle your emotions, to keep your attention and focus in one place, to eat until 80-90% full, and to eat something when you crave it and not act like you don't want it. I.E. is an education in the eating experience, focus, attention, and emotion.

Intuitive Conclusion

I have given you everything you need to know to not only understand intuitive eating, but also to practice it. Is I.E. for you? That is a question only you can answer. I.E. is great for some people, in some situations, and others need to stay away from it for now.

If you have a long way to go, or are looking for an eating lifestyle to take up long-term, I.E. is a great option. However, it isn't the diet to get you shredded the last 8-12 weeks of contest prep for a physique show. No numbers, no meal plan, just eating until you're 80-90% full, listening to your body's hunger signals and creating a satisfying eating environment.

I believe I.E. is a great form of eating to give a try. Just like IIFYM, you may like it and you may not, but you can't find what works best for you until you shop around a little bit. Here is the thing, whether you are on IIFYM, I.E. or a meal plan, you need to give it time, spend at least a couple months trying any of them before you knock them.

For myself, I believe that intuitive eating is the best way to go in terms of a way of eating that works well year-round. Counting macros all year or being on a diet plan long term can be mentally taxing - leave that to grind time when you want to make a transformation for a show or photoshoot.

IIFYM and meal plans are best for getting into incredible conditioning, but I.E. is better for lifestyle, longevity, and helps keep your focus off of food when you're not eating. I.E. is also the single most versatile form of eating, especially if you travel. When traveling, I.E. is the clear winner: meal plans suck when traveling, macros can be frustrating, but intuitive is seamless. I am sure you could understand why I.E. makes traveling less stressful.

Not having to worry about meal prep or macros while traveling allows you to focus on the traveling. There we go again, I.E. is all about focus, attention and emotional intelligence. Become an emotionally intelligent focused spirit animal of progress, with intuitive eating.

Meal Plans (Bro Diet)

When we think of diets, we normally think meal plans. Most of the world doesn't know about IIFYM, even though it's super popular in the fitness world, and intuitive eating is still in its infancy in terms of popularity and recognition, even in the fitness world.

There is one way of dieting that we are all accustomed to thinking of when it comes to bodybuilding, or just weight loss in general, and that's a "Meal Plan." Now, personally I am not a big fan of meal plans, but I am not here to be biased or to sway you towards one form of dieting or method of eating.

Meal plans do have their place, they can make life easier if done right, and they can make life dreadful if done wrong or taken up by the type of person who doesn't take well to a lot of structure. A meal plan is a pre-planned eating structure where food is measured in advance. You will normally have a set amount of meals, around 5-6 meals a day. You will eat your meals every 2.5 to 3 hours. You will also be restricting your food choices to only the meals in the meal plan. Let me give you an example of a typical meal plan of a bodybuilder:

Meal 1 (7:30 am) – *10 egg whites, one whole egg, ½ cup of oatmeal, 1 tbsp. of almond butter*

Meal 2 (10 am) – *Protein shake with a handful of spinach, 100 grams of blueberries, and a tablespoon of coconut oil.*

Meal 3 (12:30 pm) – *6 ounces of chicken breast, 8 ounces of sweet potato, 1 cup of broccoli*

Meal 4 (3:30 pm) *6 ounces of chicken breast, ½ cup of brown rice, 1 cup of broccoli*

Meal 5 (6:30 pm) *protein shake (post workout)*

Meal 6 (9:30 pm) *6 ounces of tilapia, 8 ounces of sweet potato, 1 cup of mixed veggies*

This is the stereotypical meal plan structure you will see 90% of bodybuilders following. Then there is the cult of IIFYM's that will scold them as "bro dieters" while they fit a giant melted chocolate chip cookie with ice-cream on top into their macros as their last meal.

Hey, I have done both, I have bro dieted for years as well as counted macros for years. I typically didn't fit a lot of cookies into my diet, but low fat ice-cream and a perfectly crafted chocolate protein brownie were secret weapons when contest prepping on IIFYM.

When I bro dieted for contest prep, I tended to overeat on my tablespoon of almond or peanut butter in the morning. Bro dieting has the effect of making some people crave peanut butter, and eventually be revolted by oatmeal.

You will also find yourself getting very creative with your sweet potato and rice and using zero calorie butter spray on everything. By the way, zero calorie butter spray actually has calories. Anything less than 5 calories per servings can be labeled as zero calories per the FDA. I digress, even though you just had an 'aha!' moment.

For those of you who haven't heard the fitness lingo of bro dieting, here is a little bird's eye view of this classic style of dieting. Bro meal plans are about taking every bit of processed food out of the equation and eating only whole complex carbs, lean high BV proteins, and nutrient dense fat sources like omega 3's and MCTs.

The name "bro dieting" came from the old-school bodybuilding mentality/gym fad following muscle heads like you see on the planet fitness commercials. These miraculous bro creatures believe and preach eating strictly micronutrient dense, wholesome food sources, which in their minds is completely superior to the IIFYM approach.

These are the guys that preach 6 meals a day, preach the anabolic post workout protein window, and rid the grocery store of their egg whites and oatmeal. "DISCLAIMER" I am not putting anyone down, I am joking, I love my bros, I was once a bro, being a bro is ok, just as being an avid IIFYM dude is ok.

Now, as someone who has followed flexible dieting and meal plans for contest prep, I can say that I believe meeting somewhere in the middle of "meal plan" and IIFYM works the best for me and any many others. When dieting down for a photo shoot or contest prep, I tend to eat 80-90% nutrient dense foods, but I still like to enjoy my fat free ice-cream and protein cookies.

Bro dieting isn't the only type of meal plan out there, but it is the most known and prevalent in the health and fitness industry. Ask any bodybuilder what you should do for eating and building muscle, and they will either give you the bro dieting rundown of eating every 2.5-3 hours, give you the list of bro foods, or they will tell you they count macros.

In some cases, they will tell you they don't pay attention to their diet, either they have superman genetics or they're undercover intuitive eaters, this is rare. IIFYM guys and bro dieters will always have some disagreement. The thing is, eating mostly micronutrient dense foods in a meal timing and meal frequency that works best for you does increase performance in the gym.

If you are heathier and you feel better, your workouts will be better, you will hit better numbers and get stronger. Consistently performing better will lead you to getting bigger and stronger much faster than if you were eating processed food all day.

On the opposite end of the fence, eating 100% nutrient dense whole foods takes the fun out of life, drains you, and makes you want the diet to be over so you can have variety again. I think diet plans can be very powerful and work very well for some people, but I believe the traditional bro diet should be modified to have the ability to fit occasional processed foods in. It's mentally draining to have less than 10 foods in your food arsenal to choose from, but at the same time, it's a gains killer to be eating more than 20% processed food on any given day.

Meal Prep

When we're talking about a meal plan, the most important thing to take into consideration is meal prep. At its core, meal prep is what makes a meal plan "a meal plan." You will have your meals ready to go, ready to be eaten up to a week ahead of time.

This does a few things; first of all, whenever you get

hungry for your next meal, it's just there. It is a little easier to want to eat something less nutrient dense if you have to take the time to think about it every time you go to eat. IIFYM is great but when you're just counting macros and you still have to cook or make a meal every time you're hungry, by nature you become more food focused.

When you're on a meal plan as opposed to IIFYM or I.E., you can rest assured that you are getting everything you need to build muscle and burn fat. Whether you are on a bulking meal plan or a cutting meal plan, the entire week's worth of meals is set up to carry you to that goal.

When counting macros and following I.E., you may have days where your macros are less nutrient dense. This will never happen when on a meal plan. Unless you incorporate a free meal; in other words, an unprepared meal once every week or so which is less nutrient dense, this won't happen, ever.

For some of you that's a good thing, others will feel trapped. The first thing you will need to do is stock up on **plastic food containers**. This is literally one click away on amazon, here is an amazon link to an assortment of containers for meal prep.

You can literally get them for less than a dollar per container or you could get some cool pretty colorful container for just over a $1 per container. You can get them anywhere, the Dollar Store, the grocery store, your local Wal-Mart or Target, and even your mom's kitchen.

Once you have your collection of meal prep containers, you can proudly post to Instagram saying "shit's about to get real." This is the cheapest and most helpful investment you will ever make as a bodybuilder or fitness enthusiast. The next most valuable thing would be your food scale.

Amazon has this all laid out; packages with food

containers + the food scale for around $40. Can you tell I am a big Amazon guy? That's beside the point here. What you will want to do is go buy yourself about 20 containers, a staple protein source or a few, and a few staple carb sources plus veggies and spinach. Here are the staples that work well with meal prep which most bodybuilders use.

Carb sources

1. Sweet Potato
2. Brown Rice
3. Oats

Protein Sources

1. Chicken Breast
2. Tilapia
3. Salmon
4. Tuna
5. Lean Beef
6. Lean Steak
7. Eggs
8. Whey Protein Powder

Getting in fats never seems to be too much of an issue. Anyhow, here are 2 healthy fats, one to cook with, and one to add to protein shakes.

1. Almond Butter for protein shakes
2. Coconut oil for cooking

Also, don't forget to go out and get your veggies and

spinach. I recommend getting some broccoli, medley mix, peppers, mushrooms and spinach leaves. These are all highly nutrient dense and very low calorie.

Don't forget to get some fruit, I am a big blueberry guy. Blueberries are low in a calories and very high in antioxidants, and they also provide a powerful punch of fiber. Strawberries are great as well, low calorie and very cheap when in season.

You can also add blueberries to your protein shakes or make protein pancakes and protein brownies and add blueberries and strawberries into your protein batter. Once you have your list of staple foods, stick to them. Find the best deals, which are usually at club stores like Sam's or Costco, and then get to prep.

Pick a day to go food shopping once a week, take into consideration how crowded your supermarket may be on your decided day, and commit to that day as your restock day. The goal here is to make this whole process a seamless part of your life.

Once you get all of your food on your day of choice, get it home and get to prep. Lay your 20 plastic containers out on the table - or 10, which ever fits - then get to cooking.

There are 3 ways to cook your chicken: fry it in the pan, bake or broil it in the oven, or cook it in the crockpot. I am a crockpot type of guy. You do need to take a few things into consideration when cooking chicken in different ways, things like timing and attention.

Crockpot cooking will take the longest but doesn't need any supervision. Baking and broiling is faster, whereas a crockpot takes 6-12 hours. Oven cooking only takes a few but needs to be checked and you can't leave it unattended or you will end up with no house to come back to. Frying in the pan is the fastest, you can cook pounds of chicken in an hour but it will take your undivided attention to cook it properly.

I like to really enjoy my time with the frying pan, listen to music and sing; frying pan time is my time, I don't do it often, but when I do, I enjoy it. Once the chicken is going, it's time to cut up a lot of sweet potatoes and get them started cooking. Cut up enough for at least 2-3 meals a day for your whole week.

You can either bake them, boil them on the stove or microwave them. I recommend microwaving them. All you need is a microwave friendly giant bowl and some water, wrap the top of the bowl with saranwrap to trap the heat in and put those potatoes in the microwave.

The time in the microwave depends on the amount of sweet potatoes you are cooking. You will have to experiment with this the first couple of times. It takes anywhere from 10-30 minutes depending on if you just have a few sweet potatoes or 8 in the microwave.

Once the chicken and sweet potatoes are cooking, go ahead and get a large pot ready, fill it with water and get your vegetables boiling. Vegetables don't take long at all to cook and you don't want to let them sit and boil for an hour because you will lose a lot of the nutrient make-up of the vegetables through heat. Once the vegetables come to a boil, let them boil for 10-20 minutes depending on how many vegetables you are boiling.

You don't want to overcook them, just lightly cook them. Once either the sweet potatoes or the vegetables are done, it's time to get some rice cooking; make enough for at least 1-2 meals a day or 3-4, whatever floats your boat. It's up to you whether you would like to have sweet potato as your primary source of carbs or brown rice. You can cook the rice in the microwave or just take your freshly steamed veggies out of your pot and put the rice in. I recommend Minute Maid brown rice as it cooks much more quickly than other types of rice, it's a time saver.

You can either leave the spinach completely raw as I like to do, that way it retains 100% of its nutrients, or lightly boil it with the vegetables or after with the rice. Pro tip: Line up the way you're cooking your chicken with the cooking of your carbs.

If you do cook your chicken in the crock pot, simply wait to start cooking all of your carbs until your chicken is nearly ready to be taken out. If you would like to add beef into the equation, that's as simple as putting some meat on the pan and frying it up while everything else is cooking. Yes, you can cook all of these things at once, I've done it and so have many others.

For this meal prep example, we will not be using beef or steak, only the necessities. By necessities I mean chicken, sweet potato, rice, vegetables and spinach. Once everything is done, start filling out the plastic containers with food.

I recommend cutting the sweet potatoes up into small chunks to make better use of the space in your meal prep containers. Start by placing the chopped sweet potato in each container, try to be consistent on the amount of sweet potato in each container but don't overthink it, no need to be perfect unless you are in contest prep. I recommend filling out 10 containers with sweet potato as your carb and 10 containers using brown rice as your carb.

Once the primary carb sources are laid, add your mixed veggies in, be creative you can make some meals all broccoli, other meals medley mix, some meals can be all spinach leaves and mushrooms and some meals can be an assortment of all of those food items.

Make sure that you have left enough space to lay your chicken. The amount of chicken will vary from person to person based on your body mass, goals, and gender. I recommend as a general guideline to always aim to hit your bodyweight in protein every day. Four ounces of chicken is about 24 grams of protein so you can do the math. For most women, I recommend 3-6 ounces of chicken for every meal depending on your total bodyweight.

Remember these meals are only accounting for 4 meals of your day, you will still make your breakfast and before bed meal on the spot, so you need to take into account the protein in those meals as well. However, as a general rule of thumb, if you are a 90-130 pound women, 3-4 ounces of chicken per the 4 chicken meals is ideal. If you are 140-200 lbs., 5-6 ounces of chicken per meal is a great number to aim for. For guys, I recommend 6-7 ounces per meal for 120-160lbs and 8-10 ounces per meal for dudes weighing 170-230.

Obviously, if you weigh more than that and it's all or mainly muscle, you already know how much chicken breast you need in your meals.

You can plan your meals however you want and there are several different variations of how you can set up your meal plans. Here are a few:

Meal 1- Eggs and oatmeal
Meal 2- Chicken meal
Meal 3- Chicken meal
Meal 4- Protein shake meal
Meal 5- Chicken meal
Meal 6- Chicken meal
Or for those who give no shits about breakfast
Meal 1- Chicken meal

Meal 2- Chicken meal
Meal 3- Protein shake
Meal 4- Chicken meal
Meal 5- Chicken meal
Meal 6- Protein brownie with sugar free syrup and fat free whip crème, feel free to add blueberries into the mix.
Or even for the people who want to be rebellious.
Meal 1- Protein Pancake with sugar free syrup + oatmeal with a dab of sugar free syrup
Meal 2- Chicken meal
Meal 3- Chicken meal
Meal 4- Chicken meal
Meal 5- Chicken meal
Meal 6- Protein cookie heated, with fat free ice-cream on top (only one serving)

There are several different ways you can do a meal plan; you don't have to have protein shakes at all, but I believe variety is key. The classic 'eating 6 meals a day of the same exact thing every day' is a recipe for failure. Variety is the spice of life even if you're on a meal plan.

When I say chicken meal, I mean chicken, your carb source and your veggies. You can also switch out a few chicken meals for beef meals or fish meals.

This will all come down to what works best for you, your budget, and how much time you're willing to put into meal prep. The more diverse, the more prep time. IIFYM and meal plans, contrary to popular belief, are really not much different at all. This is why I shake my head when I see IIFYM guys battling it out with meal plan guys. We are all doing the same thing, just strutting it in a different way.

Meal Plans (The Bodybuilders Diet)

Ever since Arnold become the King of aesthetics and even before, bodybuilders have been following meal plans. You could say that meal plans were the original IIFYM, except classic bodybuilders were religious about only fitting in certain foods into their meal plans.

Two big things that carried the art of bodybuilding to where it is today are highly structured meal plans and crazy intense super high volume workouts. Eating these meal plans and taking the human body to an elite state represents a level that only a few will ever see themselves get to because very few will ever have the discipline, devotion, and dedication to get there.

Most IFBB pro bodybuilders still follow meal plans religiously; only a few of them follow flexible dieting/ IIFYM. You will see more natural bodybuilders following IIFYM while IFBB and NAPA bodybuilders tend to opt for the meal plans.

The meal plan can be looked at in many ways; to a classic bodybuilder sticking to a meal plan and not going over, to the IIFYM side, there is the same dedication and loyalty to what got them to where they are. Here is the thing, if something is working for you why change it? If IIFYM works for you, keep counting macros, if meal plans work for you, stay on a meal plan!

There is some method to the bro madness - if you read the first section of the book and learned about the molecular science, you know that over time eating nutrient dense food over nutrient dead food will make a huge difference in your physique, health and lifespan.

I love IIFYM and coach most of my clients using IIFYM, but the problem with the younger generation is the fact that they look at the classic "bro dieters" like they're ignorant. They're not ignorant, they're a different generation. Both generations could learn from each other if they could only lose the ego a little. I think a lot of classic bodybuilders can learn to be less robotic about dieting, and modern day IIFYM guys can learn to stop fitting so much shit into their macros.

Bodybuilders have built beautiful physiques for a very long time using strict meal plans, so we can't disregard this classic way of thinking and eating simply because there are newer, more glamorous ways to diet.

Meal Plan vs. IIFYM

On no, did I just go there? Yep, I went there. Let me start this unbiased dispute off by saying that IIFYM and meal plans are one in the same. When you diet on a meal plan, the meal plan is based on hitting consistent macros.

One way that meal plans take the cake over IIFYM is the fact that you prepare all of your meals ahead of time, either once or twice a week, and then you don't have to think about food at all.

Once you have all of your meals prepped, which takes only a couple of hours once or twice a week, you don't need to think about numbers, hitting numbers, making sure you hit macros by the end of the day, or making sure you don't go over macros.

You don't have to worry about numbers or focus on food at all, you simply eat the meals you have laid out for yourself and go on about your day. So you have more food choice freedom when counting macros, but at the same time you have to think about food all day, and count numbers all day.

Would you rather have little structure with your diet, but be calculating macros all day to hit your numbers or have a set meal plan where you stick to only that meal plan, no numbers, no counting? You see, counting macros makes you more food focused, meal plans restrict your food choices.

Being food focused and restricting one's self can both have negative effects on your relationship to food. I think having staple carbs sources, protein sources and fat sources is the way to go 100%; this structure is a product of meal planning.

I also believe that you need to not be overly restrictive when you want something that may not be on your meal plan. I like to look at a meal plan as a template; you can have 2-3 complex carb sources to alternate between to keep things from getting stale, 2-3 protein sources, 2-3 fat sources, and the option to alternate between protein shake, protein brownie or protein pancake, with the occasional protein cookie.

Now, in my opinion, this is how a meal plan ought to be designed. All 6 of your meals are set but if you want to swap out meal 6 from being a protein shake to being a protein brownie one day, do it. If you want to swap out meal one from being egg whites and oatmeal to being a protein pancake with sugar free syrup and blueberries, do it.

Contrary to popular belief, you actually easily eat out with your friends on a meal plan.

If meal 5 is chicken, sweet potato and broccoli, I hate to be the bearer of bad news, but you could have eaten that with your friends at just about anywhere. When you go out to eat for one of your meals, just make sure to tell them no butter, steam the veggies, no brown sugar and butter on the sweet potato (instead use Splenda, yes that tastes great when you're dieting).

Also make sure that whether you get steak, fish or chicken that it isn't cooked in any high fat oils or butter unless you purposely want to get in some fat on that particular meal, in that case go for it. You can basically do the same thing with macros that you can do with a meal plan, which is why I look at them both as pretty much the same.

Macros and meal plans are like father and son. Either of them can get you to your goals, but a meal plan can beat counting macros any day if it is put together correctly.

In-between IIFYM & I.E.

I find myself calling a meal plan the in-between of IIFYM and intuitive in some ways. When following I.E., there is no food focus at all. IIFYM is arguably the most food focused form of eating of meal plans, IIFYM and I.E. When eating intuitively, you're not tracking anything, with a meal plan you are not tracking as strictly as on macros, but you still have some food focus, just not a lot.

The Hybrid: Meal Plans + IIFYM + I.E.

What if it was possible to be on a hybrid meal plan that incorporated properties of I.E. & IIFYM? What if you could be on a meal plan that allowed you to eat 6 meals a day with high quality sources of protein, carbs and fat that was also flexible and intuitive?

You can, yes, this is real life. When you're reading this subchapter, turn on some cinematic trance music to allow the proper brain absorption of such a game changing, revolutionary, innovative idea! Let me show you how this would look.

Eat until 80-90% full if you feel full before you finish you stop eating. This goes for all 6 meals.

Meal 1- Eggs and oatmeal, or protein pancake & wholegrain waffles, or chicken & egg & whole grain waffles, or steak & egg with a whole grain pancake.

Meal 2- Chicken meal or 90% lean beef meal (using sweet potato as carb source or brown rice, or couscous).

Meal 3- Chicken meat or fish meal or Tofu meal (using vegetable medley, or green beans or spinach, or cucumber and lettuce salad. Pro tip: Use fat free ranch or other types of dressing. Also check the carbs, there are some very tasty low calorie salad dressings that allow salads to remain low calorie.

Meal 4- Protein shake meal, or protein brownie with high protein, low fat Greek yogurt and some almond butter, or protein cookie with coconut oil and fat free syrup, or low-fat ice-cream.

Meal 5- Chicken meal, or mixed steak & chicken meal (using whole grain, lower calorie burrito wraps).

Meal 6- Chicken meal, or reduced fat pork meal, or cottage cheese meal, or lentils meal using quinoa or soba noodles or Edamame (which is a high plant protein green been), or even navy beans, which are so high in protein that you will need less of a protein source for this meal.

If you know what your numbers are, you can create a meal plan with enough options to keep you going for a very long time. We look at meal plans the wrong way; we look at meal plans like they're only this bland bro dieting eating tactic that only classic bro bodybuilders use.

If you aren't trying to get stage lean (sub 6% body fat),

then there is no need to be on the needle when it comes to macros, meals and food weight, so why stress it? It's a total and 100% myth that eating only "bro foods" will yield you the best gains. In fact, having a wider variety of meal options in your meal plan will allow you to have more diversity in your nutrients, which could be healthier then only having 2 carb sources and 2-3 protein sources as your staple choices.

When it comes to eating structure and dieting, you have got to remember that this whole thing is highly psychological. The whole reason that we have intuitive, IIFYM and meal plans is because we are all so different.

Each one of us think very differently, have very different goals, have very different habitual conditionings, and have different relationships with food, etc. What I am trying to do here is get you to think outside the box a little, forget there was ever a box, and construct your own box.

Some of you won't be efficient on a 100% IIFYM based diet, or a 100% I.E. based protocol, or even a 100% meal plan structured diet. Some of you will want to create a hybrid plan because of your mix of all of the differentiating factors I just mentioned. Extremes are never healthy in life, never, ever.

Meal Plan Companies

If you have a little extra money to invest in your diet and physique, you can now hire a meal plan company to build you a meal plan with macros, diverse food choices, the whole shebang. Just like that hybrid meal plan example I just showed you, you can basically find meal plan catering companies that can build you just about any type of meal plan.

There are even some meal prep companies that create meal plans personalized to your exact macros for the day, topped off with macro friend's cake, cookies and ice cream when you want it. I really believe this is the future - <u>I am saying this right now, Saturday, June 18th, 2016, that meal prep companies are going to be taking over the dieting industry in less than 5 years, mark my words.</u>

Once these companies grow bigger, price goes down, and more exposure comes out, getting your meals for the day and week personally delivered to your house, hitting your macros with whatever foods you want. Oh yeah, that will make life easier.

We live in a world where time and convenience is our most valuable commodity. That's why meal plan companies will blow up; that why Uber does so well, and that's why you're reading this book. You may be able to build a meal plan and meal prep it every week, but what if you could have a drone deliver your meals for the week, prepped, tasty and ready to eat?

You may be able to get all of the info in this book scattered across google but with a completely different context. But you may never find all that, and it may take you years to do it. This is the same reason that I believe in the battle of dieting and building the physique, meal plans will always win the popular vote. They're the least time consuming, the least food focused and the most convenient. I rest my case.

Going Past Bro

When we think of meal plans, we think of chicken, fish, egg whites, broccoli, sweet potatoes, brown rice and oatmeal. We also think of eating 6 meals a day, every 2.5

to 3 hours. Here's the thing, a meal plan can be built using any food sources and any amount of meals and timing.

The important thing is that you do have an actual structured plan where you have set out meals for the next three days to a week. You need high quality sources of protein, high quality sources of complex carbs, as well as micronutrient dense carbs like broccoli and spinach leaves. Lastly, you need to make sure you get high quality sources of fats, i.e. nuts, coconut oils, nut oils and fish oils.

Whether you are following paleo, vegan, tropical or bro, you can create a meal plan in any way you want. What I want you to realize is that meal plans don't have to be these bland bro diets that only classic bodybuilders follow, and not all meal plans are cookie cutters.

Now, obviously if you want a meal plan customized to you, you will need to build it yourself or hire a coach to build it. Meal plans are templates with guidelines; the structure, types of food, timing and frequency should be completely predicated on when you like to eat, what foods you enjoy, how often you like to eat, etc.

That is how to create a meal plan that will work for you, personally. Create a meal plan around you, yourself and your life. Don't create your life around your meal plan, that is the problem with some meal plans. They aren't created around one's life, one is trying to balance life with the meal plan, therefore making the meal plan unsustainable.

Cons of Meal Plans

- *"The bro stigma, and the idea that all meal plans are bro."* If we look at the original bodybuilding meal plan, the bro meal plan, it's not flexible. This means you will eat the same food, every day, for the duration of the meal plan.

Yep, if you ask some innocent bystander at the gym that just so happens to be on the gear, the juicy juice, the shit, he may just spout out how many egg whites he eats in the morning. "YOU NEED THE BROTIEN BROOOO." All of those egg whites (12-20) with a large cup of plain oats, and a scoop of peanut butter, maybe. That is the breakfast of the champions, the breakfast of the bropions.

Next, this habitual machine of destruction is going to tell you how he's eating every 2.5 hours on the dot, because the body can't absorb more than 50 grams of protein at a time, right babe?

Only complex carbs (in other words not intuitive eating) like sweet potato and brown rice with the protein packed chicken meals that are consumed every 2.5 hours. You have to keep the metabolism burning in high gear with those frequent meals of the bropions.

Once you finish your workout, you must consume a whey protein shake or you will lose all of your gains and become sterile. You can basically eat as many complex carbs as you want because the body will use is to fuel the muscles. But if you take on just one meal of complex carbs and eat skittles, your body will secrete insulin and you will gain fat.

Simple sugars automatically turn to fat because, well, because science. Must do your cardio before you eat breakfast, otherwise no fat will be burned my bro, then you must eat egg whites. You must have this breakfast immediately after your fasted cardio or your metabolism will stop working. The more meat you eat, the faster your metabolism. Eat 6-8 meals a day and twice your bodyweight in protein and you will look like me in months.

That's right, you will gain 30 pounds of solid muscle in less than 3 months. Now hand over the $300, my knowledge is not free. Oh, one more thing, never eat carbs at night, you will store all of them as fat. **(Disclaimer)** Everything I just said was bullshit.

This is why you don't run up to the biggest guy at the gym and ask him for a meal plan to get like him. I understand if you are new to this, but be smart. Be smart with your money, and be smart with your beliefs.

If something sounds too good to be true it is probably "bro science." Bro science is pumped up bullshit using studies and statistics that promote lies about diet and training and give young and impressionable physique builders false expectations.

With meal plans, we will always have the bro stigma. This is really nothing more than a stigma, it's not real. The problem is that a lot of us think of a meal plan as "a bro diet" and for that reason we will never go on any sort of meal plan because of our own ego.

This was me for a while after I discovered IIFYM, as many other young physique builders. Meal plans can be awesome, so don't think about them with such a closed minded view. Meal plans may have been just "the bro diet" before but not anymore, not after what you have just read. Meal plans are the father of IIFYM.

There is more to meal plans than bropion bullshit. There is the profound ability to build a meal plan around anything you can wrap you're head around.

Meal plans aren't for everyone. Some people just don't do well with that much structure. Structured meal timing, food prep, selective food types, etc. If you are the type of person who doesn't like structure, bad news: you can't get more structured than a meal plan. If you think counting macros is structured, meal plans dictate the times you eat, and your food types, not just your macro numbers.

- If too much structure stresses you out, makes life harder on you, makes you feel like you can't deal, don't go on a meal plan. You need to opt more towards intuitive eating or possibly IIFYM. At the end of the day, all 3 ways of eating can produce great results and can be great for lifestyle. The issue that a lot of us are missing is that, while every form of dieting can work, you need to find the form that will work, for you, today.

- Meal plans can work year-round, but I wouldn't ask anyone to follow a set meal plan all year. I wouldn't consider a meal plan to be a way of eating that you can follow the rest of your life. You can follow the structure of a meal plan, meal prep, etc. But at some point, it should become more intuitive, at which point the meal plan is now intuitive eating.

Meal plans are great for dieting down for photo shoots, shows, or learning how to structure your macros, meal timing and meal prep, but when we are talking about 24/7/365, meal plans get old. Even the idea of being on a meal plan gets old. Sometimes it's nice not to have a plan. Sometimes it's nice to go on vacation and not pre plan anything you eat.

Personally, I am not a huge planning guy, so I am about 40% intuitive, 40% IIFYM and 20% meal plan. Preparing the chicken and carb sources is a great practice to have all of the time, but I don't think the entirety and structure of a meal plan is needed year-round. Once you have been on a meal plan for so long, it becomes intuitive, that will just happen

I would go so far as to say that being on a meal plan year round isn't mentally healthy; you shouldn't be thinking about food, food prep, and plastic food containers all the time. You should be living life, focusing on the rest of life. While what we eat and how much is important, 25% or more of our life shouldn't be spent thinking about and preparing food, unless we are in the culinary arts.

You don't want to be that guy at your friend's wedding that can't eat cake, or any of the other delicious food at the wedding. You don't want to be that guy that has to pull out a plastic container with chicken and sweet potato at your uncle's family grill out. You definitely don't want to be the guy that goes out on a date to a restaurant that doesn't fit into your meal plan and find yourself not eating on a first date. You could have had a second date. Who knows, that could have been your future ex-girlfriend, you definitely missed out, bro.

Now, we all get into situations where we are dieting for a show or photo shoot and can't indulge in grandma's cooking or our best friend's wedding food. You know as well as I do, if you're dieting for something important, sacrifices must be made. If you aren't dieting for anything pressing, don't be a bro, enjoy yourself and be human.

- If your relationship with food is terrible, you do not need to go on any sort of meal plan, probably not even macros. You need a better relationship with food through intuitive eating. Meal plan is restrictive in nature.

When you already have a wounded relationship with food, you don't know when to stop eating or you don't eat; you need to heal that relationship as priority #1. Restriction of food variety tends to worsen problems of bad relationships with food because of the nature of reverse psychology.

When you restrict yourself more and more, it causes you to want what you aren't getting; the more you deprive yourself, the more you crave the things you are depriving yourself of. This builds an intense emotional craving towards things that you can't eat on your meal plan. Two things are bound to happen: either you fall off of your meal plan and binge, or you hit your goal, finish your meal plan, then binge on the things you deprived yourself of until you have gained back all the weight you worked so hard to lose.

The same applies to hard gainers who are trying to gain weight. If you are a hard gainer and you are trying to force yourself to stick to a high calorie gainer meal plan with only complex carbs and lean proteins, you are apt to fail. For hard gainers, getting enough calories from whole foods without feeling like you're going to puke all of the time is nearly impossible.

When trying to pack on the weight, sticking to a whole food meal plan may cause you to eventually go back to your old habits of eating random bags of potato chips and the occasional protein shake. As a hard gainer, eat all of your "bro food," but make it a point to enjoy some ice cream, pizza and candy on occasion.

If you are a serious automorphic hard gainer, you may even need to eat ice-cream and peanut butter every day to pack in the calories. Coconut oil can also be a great gainer; low volume, high calorie. The fact is, either way that you look at it, some people just won't do well on meal plans, it's important to know if you are one of those people, and also to come to terms with that fact and follow a protocol that will allow you to move forward.

- Meal plans are nearly impossible to manage when traveling. IIFYM is tough when traveling but meal plans are a no go. You can't stick on a meal plan when eating hotel food and eating out at restaurants on the road.

If you are only away from home for 3 days to a week, you could prepare all of your meals and take them with you, but would your hotel room have a big enough fridge? Better get an Airbnb with a normal sized fridge everywhere you go.

The bigger issue here is that when you are traveling for more than one week, you will run out of food prep. Since you're traveling, not even the food prep companies will be able to keep up with you. It is possible; IFFBB pro bodybuilders and Mr. Olympia actually do meal prep out of hotel rooms for much longer than a week straight.

Here is the thing, they have help. They basically have a portable kitchen with them at all times, as well as a helping hand to prepare all of their food. Want to carry around a microwave, 2 mini fridges, some electric cookers and a shaker cup with a bag of whey? Minus the bag of whey and shaker cup, it's not really practical for most of us to carry around a kitchen in our car. And if we are flying, there is no way that's getting through security.

If you're not a pro bodybuilder, and you don't make your living from fitness, even the thought of trying to meal prep and stay on a meal plan while on the road is a buzz kill.

To be honest with you, I make a living from fitness, and I would still never try to meal prep while traveling. Counting macros while traveling is the way to go if in contest prep or getting ready for a photo shoot, but if you're not getting ready for anything where you need to have your physique dialed in, do yourself a favor and go intuitive while on the road.

Meal Plan Pros

Meal plans may seem all negative as they catch a lot of fire from the IIFYM-ers and the intuitive eaters. But despite all this, meal plans can be amazing tools and ways of eating.

There are many ways that meal plans are far superior to IIFYM and I.E. If done right, meal plans can just about work for anyone; anyone that does well with a good amount of structure. Let's take a look at all of the things that help meal plans to stand out as a dieting method.

- First of all, meal plans are literally the most accurate form of dieting possible for the contest prepper or the person who is four weeks out from a photo shoot. Counting macros is accurate but you still have a slight difference in food from day to day, and no meal timing. The bro diet may not be fun to do for more than a couple of months, but utilizing the methods of the classic bro for 2-3 months to really dial in the physique for a show photoshoot allows you to be 100% accurate. With this form of dieting you will have the least fluctuation with weigh-ins day to day, the most linear weight loss, and you will ensure that you won't starve.

   When getting really lean for contest prep, cookies and ice-cream aren't our friends the last month of our contest prep diets. When you are already on low macronutrients and you're eating considerably less food than your body is comfortable with, the last thing you need to do is try fitting a cookie into your meal plan or macros. When your leptin levels are low and you are hungry all of the time, salad and vegetables are you're best friends. As well as all of the bro foods.

I recommend being as close as possible to eating 100% clean the last month of a diet leading up to a physique contest or photo shoot. The closer you get to your moment, the more control you want to have on how your physique looks from day to day. Water weight, muscle fullness, hunger, quality of workouts, mood - these are the most important things to focus on when approaching the moment where your physique will be on display.

The best way to stay happy, somewhat satiated, full and dry looking, and hitting high quality workouts is to feed your body only valuable calories. When your macros and overall calories are low, you can't afford to be throwing any of them away.

Fitting crap into your meal plan or macros when at super low body fat levels and dieting on super low calories is actually a bit dangerous. It's already super unhealthy when dieting to stay lean; you start fitting processed food in until you're at poverty macros and you will end up with a short term nutrient deficiency. You will be starving all of the time, sleepless, and your workouts will suffer.

For all of these reasons, I believe that a meal plan is the way to go when it comes to the final stages of a contest prep. I tend to diet 20+ weeks for contest prep and about 8 to 12 weeks for photo shoots, and I will say from my 6+ years of experience following different eating protocols for contest prep and photo shoot prep, that IIFYM and intuitive are great until the last couple months of prep.

That last 8 weeks of any sort of prep need to be the weeks where you dial your body into shape, which requires a low margin of error in the diet in order to see the weight loss trending day by day, week by week. At the end of the day no dieting protocol will ever be able to hold a candle to accuracy of a proper meal plan during the last couple weeks of a physique prep. Meal prep is kind when it comes to accuracy for contest prep.

- Meal plans will always win when it comes to convenience. When we talk about macros over meal plans, in terms of convenience it's very difficult to argue that IIFYM can even compete with meal plans. We can even completely outsource our meal plans.

So, basically if you know your macros and what you like to eat, granted you have the money, your diet plan and meal prep can be 100% outsourced. Even if you do everything yourself, like most of us, it only takes one trip to the grocery store and a couple of hours spent on food prep to have a successful meal plan set up.

If you have a mentally demanding job, counting and fitting in macros may be something you would rather not deal with. It may be much less mental strain on you to just have a set meal plan with a couple of choices for each meal.

- If you are one of those people (like me), who tends to overthink everything, a meal plan can really be a time and attention saver. I have ADD and I am a creative and I like numbers. It's easy to find myself making strange creations and getting completely carried away inventing some extravagant food item that fits into my remaining macros for the day.

Spending your creativity on some sort of macronutrient masterpiece can be fun, but most of us don't really have time to be playing macro chef four hours a day. We need to keep our focus on our actual life; eating is not life, it's only part of life.

Our focus needs to be on the people that are important to us; our passions, our careers, just life. The biggest mistake that I, and many other physique builders have made, is becoming overly obsessed with food and thinking that's ok.

If you are spending over 20% of your day thinking about food, or preparing food on a daily basis, you need to reevaluate your eating protocol and your relationship with food.

- Meal plans present the unique proposition of being the most consistent way to diet conveniently. Meal plans are easy to make, versatile when need be, the most accurate form of dieting when desired, plus they offer a way to teach us discipline.

With all of these 'relationship to food' arguments and 'IIFYM vs. meal plan arguments,' it's easy to forget the amount of discipline and devotion you create around a meal plan and how that helps you grow as a person. We aren't just born with discipline, we aren't just born devoted to things, and we aren't just born dedicated to things. We don't just have will power, we have to build it.

Some may argue that the millennial generation and the up and coming digital natives are brought up with a lower threshold for pain when it comes to consistently putting in the hard work. Work smarter not harder, right? Well, the problem is we are all trying to work smarter. What it comes down to is the person who is the hardest working person who also works smarter, will win.

Eating on a meal plan takes actual planning, food prep, and being consistent with whole foods, meal timing, etc. Some people that will argue that they have bad relationships to food and can't count macros or go on meal plans are really just lazy people who have never wanted to put effort into anything.

Yep, I could very damn well be talking to you. Good news, it's not too late to devote yourself to building your physique, eating better and living a healthy life. It's not too late to dedicate yourself to becoming a badass, and leaving behind your "sorryassness."

Meal plans teach structure, timing, preparation, consistency, and accuracy. If you're one of those people that's looked at the Mediterranean diet, paleo, vegan, been intrigued by intermittent fasting and secretly wants to look and feel better, listen closely. WAKE THE FUCK UP, stop thinking, stop window shopping, stop teasing the idea of changing, and CHANGE!!!

Go to the store and get some chicken breast, eggs, egg whites, sweet potatoes, brown rice, spinach leaves, veggies, fruit fish and lean beef. Come back home and prep some meals. Don't worry about macros, don't worry about anything else, learn how to eat like someone who cares about their mind, body and life.

If you read this book and continue to sit on your ass and feel sorry for yourself, it is your fault, it's on you, and I won't feel sorry for you, not one bit of sorrow. We all at some point in our life read some book, saw some fitness model, looked at the mirror and broke it, were told by our doctor we had to eat differently or we would die, couldn't take being bullied anymore.

We all reach that point where enough is enough and we pull the plug and jump into the pool, holding nothing back. Every single one of us that made that decision changed forever. We took that trip to the grocery store and got our protein, carb, and fat sources. We got a gym membership and watched a lot of YouTube videos on how to bench press, squat, deadlift, overhead press, and build a workout plan. We prepped more meals, more chicken breast meals, more fish, protein shakes, fresh fruits and veggies. We put in the days at the gym, we put in the days eating the "bro foods," and we devoted ourselves to changing from the inside out.

For me, I went on my first "bro diet" meal plan at age 14 and competed in my first bodybuilding show at 15. It changed my life forever. When I started lifting weights at 12 I was 140 pounds, 5 foot 4 inches, and about 25-28% body fat with 11.5 inch arms. In 3 years, by 15-years-old, I had learned everything I could about meal prep, dieting and training.

This is when I dieted down for my first bodybuilding show using the "bro meal plan." Chicken, broccoli, egg whites and oatmeal, that's pretty much all I ate. I competed back then at around 10% body fat, 5 foot 5 inches with 14.5 inch arms at around 156 pounds stage weight. This was the first time I ever saw my abs.

• If you are a beginner in the lifting, bodybuilding, physique building and strength building world, the bro meal plan is a great foundation. For newcomers, we either learn how to flexible diet, or bro diet from the beginning.

While I think it's important to learn and understand both counting macros and meal plans, I believe the eating clean, meal plan approach is a better foundation than just fitting in macros and counting numbers. While it's important to learn how many grams of fat, carb, and protein you personally need to gain weight, maintain weight, and lose weight, it is equally if not more important to learn proper nutrition.

There is no replacement for learning how to plan your bodybuilding meals, meal prep, meal timing, and the discipline it takes to eat like a physique building machine. We must learn macros, and we must also learn "bro nutrition." Then we can begin our journey with a strong foundation.

It's easy when starting to not pay attention to your diet, or eat a lot of shit. The basics of eating clean, complex carbs, fresh veggies, fresh leaves, high BV proteins, omega 3, omega 6, and MCT's are more important than hitting your macros. The kid that starts out simply hitting macros with no regard to micronutrients, energy balance, and the long-term effects that different types of fat, carbs and protein have on the body, is going to make much less progress as compared to the kid that follows a nutrient dense meal plan.

Remember, macros (numbers that is) are all that matters in a short term, calories in vs. calories out mentality, but that's as far as it goes. When we look at performance, the types of carbs, fat and protein matter almost as much as the amount of them you are eating.

While you could eat all of your carbs in pop tarts and doughnuts instead of sweet potatoes, brown rice and oatmeal, you wouldn't want to. The thing is, performance is directly related to what you eat and your overall health is directly related to how you eat.

You could get shredded on just pop tarts and protein shakes, it's a fact, you could but you will feel like shit. Your workouts would be shit, you would never be able to shit, and your energy would rise and plummet all day. Also, you would eventually become a diabetic.

You can't perform well in the gym if you have no energy. If you can't perform well in the gym, you won't build much muscle because you won't be motivated to lift much weight or do many sets.

When your energy is down your mood will also be down; this takes you out of a muscle building environment. Burning fat while eating shit is even worse because your body needs all the nutrients it can get while on a caloric deficit.

Not eating enough nutrients while dieting is a sure way to lose muscle. Over the years, nutrient deficiencies bring a whole host of sickness and diseases with them. After all, just by breathing air you're taking in toxins - we need antioxidants to fight the free radicals we consume by breathing.

You could build muscle and get shredded all while eating pop tarts, potato chips, fried chicken and fried fish. You could get results that way, but you will also be speeding up your aging process, hurting your metabolism over time, killing your hormones over time, making yourself less happy than you could be, and feeling much less energetic than you could feel.

Meal Plan Conclusion

I will end this section by saying that meal plans are nothing more than a structured way of pre planning your food while knowing that your macros should always be a part of your meal plan. Also, that a meal plan has no boundaries; it doesn't have to be bro, or 6 meals a day.

You can develop a meal plan off of completely odd ball sources of foods as long as they meet your needs and lead you towards your fat loss or muscle gain goals. You could eat two big meals in a day, one at 3pm and another at 9pm, and intermittent fast from waking to 2:45 pm. You could plan all of your meals to be from McDonalds and Wendy's; yes, you can eat healthy at fast food restaurants.

If you wanted to you could make a meal plan using the Mediterranean diet foods, the tropical diet foods, the paleo diet foods, the vegan diet, the man on the moon diet, the tren diet, the plutonium diet. OK, those last three weren't real, if you even for one second wondered if they were real, allow one smack on the bottom from your significant other.

I will tell you one thing; a lot of those bros at the gym are on the tren diet. Seriously though, a meal plan is nothing more than a consistent way of eating regarding food variety and timing.

The reason I see meal plans kicking I.E.'s and IIFYM's asses is the fact they can be almost as versatile as IIFYM and they are more accurate then both IIFYM and intuitive. They are also the most convenient form of dieting and teach more discipline, devotion, and dedication than I.E. or IIFYM.

But meal plans aren't for everybody; some who are complete free spirits at nature just don't do well with the idea of planning anything. Others need to nourish their relationship with food before counting macros or building a meal plan.

At the end of the day, whether you choose IIFYM, I.E. or a meal plan is dependent on you - your lifestyle and your psychology at this current moment in time. You may even use all three methods of eating at different points in your life as your relationship to food changes, as your perception of these three forms of dieting changes, and as your goals change over time.

There is no best way of eating, no best way to get shredded, and no best way to build muscle when it comes to your dieting protocol. The only "best diet" is the diet that works the best for you at this moment.

SECTION 3

MEAL TIMING & DIETING SUBCATEGORIES

Besides the three ways we can program our food, there are a couple of ways we can program our meal timing and meal frequency. There are also many different food variety plans ranging from the McDonalds diet to the tropical diet.

Obviously, we already know about the bro diet. With three different major ways to program your diet, several ways to program your meal timing and frequency, and endless food variety plans, the possibilities are endless. Let's start by discussing food timing and frequency.

Eating every 2.5 to 3 hours for hard gainers.

Let me start off by saying what eating every 2.5 to 3 hours doesn't do for you:

1. It doesn't affect your metabolism.

2. It doesn't help you build more muscle than eating less frequently.

3. It isn't better than eating 3-4 meals a day.

Your metabolism is dictated by many things, body mass, muscle mass, lifestyle, gender, genetics, etc. However, one thing that doesn't affect your metabolism is meal timing. Yep I said it, and meal timing doesn't have anything to do with your basal metabolic rate.

Eating less frequently throughout the day won't drop your metabolism, and eating more frequently throughout the day won't elevate your metabolism. It's all about your total macronutrient and caloric intake for the day.

If you eat 300 carbs, 60 grams of fat and 150 grams of protein, whether you eat those macros spread out through 6 meals or 2, it's still going be 300C, 60F, 150P. My point is, don't stress about food timing when it comes to your metabolism.

When it comes to eating every 3 hours to absorb protein, this is also bullshit. Your protein intake for the day is what counts; your body will adapt to whatever food timing you throw at it. It really doesn't matter all that much when you eat your protein, as long as your hit your target protein numbers. Eating 6 meals a day simply isn't superior to eating 3-4 meals a day for any reason. All supporting reasons are "bro science" myths.

However, eating more frequently will allow a hard gainer to throw down more food. If you're a hard gainer, it can be really difficult to eat large amounts of food at one sitting. I don't recommend intermittent fasting or eating 1-2 meals a day for any serious ectomorphs.

What do I a mean by serious ectomorphs? I am talking about the guys that eat 3000 calories a day and can't gain any weight. I am talking about the people who need 4000-6000 calories a day to be in a caloric surplus, and who tend to have small appetites. If you get full on 8 ounces of chicken and a cup of rice, then there is absolutely no way you can try eating 1-3 big meals, or you will feel like a balloon all of the time and get sick when you work out.

Eating more meals will allow time for some of the food you're eating to settle and digest so that you can throw down more food. Hard gainers need to eat like beasts to gain mass, period. Eat your 5-6 meals a day, hit your bodyweight in protein, keep eating carbs until you see GAINS, and do this until you're actually gaining weight, even if it's one pound per month.

After you have eaten all of the complex carbs and good fats, and hit your protein numbers for the day, eat some damn ice-cream. If you want, eat pizza, a doughnut; you need to get those calories in my skinny friend. Use the bro diet tactics to your advantage but at the end of the day, throw the calories in.

For someone who has the metabolic capacity to burn 5,000 to 6,000 calories a day eating 1,000 to even 2,000 calories of processed food, one day isn't going to hurt them. The people that are hurting themselves are the people who eat 3,000 calories of processed food with a metabolic capacity genetically able to handle around 2,500 calories.

This person will probably end up a diabetic with many diseases by the time they are 50. So, what I am saying is eating every 2.5 to 3 hours and eating 6 or more meals a day should be tools of the hard gainer. I can't recommend eating that frequently to anyone with a higher appetite and a slower metabolism.

Eating every 3 hours is bad for easy gainers.

If you gain weight easily and lose weight slowly, I am right there by your side. We tend to have more cravings and have a bigger appetite, but ironically will become obese if we eat 3/4 as much food as a true hard gainer eats every day.

We need bigger meals later in the day in order to feel more satisfied. I don't recommend eating over 3-4 meals for anyone who can gain weight easily. I will even go so far as to say that for easy gainers, the best thing to do is to either skip breakfast, or eat light, and eat a medium sized lunch.

I recommend a large salad for lunch. Eat as light in regards to calories until late evening, the more calories and macronutrients we easy gainers can save for later on in the day the bigger meals we can eat in the evening and at night. I recommend your biggest meal being at night so that you go to bed feeling full and satisfied.

So, small or no breakfast, low calorie + high volume lunch, large dinner and large before-bed meal. For the last meal before bed I recommend having something you enjoy. You shouldn't eat super high volume but have something tasty and satisfying, and always eat until 80-90% full, always.

I think intermittent fasting, which I discuss in the next section, is a blessing for any easy gainer or for people who are looking to stay lean year around, because it allows you to focus on your day; no food focus, and then you get to eat like a king later on in the evening. The I.E. protocol works very well for most endomorphic, easy gainer types. It works great for me, and it can work great for any other easy gainer who either wants to get shredded or maintain a lean physique.

Intermittent Fasting (I.F.)

Intermittent Fasting is a very popular meal timing protocol that uses fasting windows as opposed to full on fasting. Popular to contrary belief, intermittent fasting doesn't have any profound fat burning, muscle building or super health benefits.

Instead, I.F. is highly predicated on psychology and satiety. There are many different ways to I.F. but in the fitness world, it means holding off on eating from wake-up until a specific time of the day. The amount of time you fast is going to be determined by your precise tolerance to fasting.

The more frequently you are used to eating, the harder it will be to fast for any amount of time. I.F. does work, it does have a lot of benefits, and there are many different ways that you can use I.F., I am going to explain everything to you right now.

Easing into I.F.

One cannot simply go straight from eating 6 meals a day directly to waking and intermittently fasting until 4pm. What I suggest is to start by reducing your breakfast on the first couple of days up to a week. After a week, go ahead and delay or eliminate breakfast.

I suggest drinking 1-2 liters of water with lemon juice

and even water flavoring if you want. This will give you some energy, wake you up and set the mood for your day. If you are a coffee drinker like me, you never stop drinking coffee and need creamer. I use I creamer which is fat free, sugar free (Coffee Mate).

When intermittent fasting, I only use about 3-5 servings of creamer. Technically, you're now eating some calories, but the whole point of I.F. is to save the bulk of calories for later in the day and not completely just balls to the wall fast with only water. Once you have gotten your morning down to just water, or coffee and water, throw your first meal off for 2 hours.

Congratulations, you have just created a 2-hour intermittent fasting window. Take anywhere from one to three weeks to get accustomed to that 2-hour window. Once you feel like you are used to the 2-hour fasting window, jump up to a 4-hour fasting window, no food for the first 4 hours.

At this point, you will probably have a little more difficulty adjusting to the larger fasting window. I like to introduce some green tea or a low fat chia latte. Find your favorite green or herbal tea, add a spoonful of stevia or Splenda, and there is another tasty beverage to suit your habitual need to be putting something to your mouth.

Yes, just as smokers are habitually used to the ritual of putting the cigarette in their mouth and smoking it, we are all wired to eat the way we have habitually eaten. By supplementing the food for flavored water, coffee and green tea, we are replacing calories with liquids to keep us satiated and energetic until our intermittent fast ends.

Let's say for example you wake up at 7am. At this point you are now fasting until 11am. I recommend holding the 4 hour fast for about 2 weeks, then starting to change that first meal. You're first meal should be a high volume, high protein, low calorie meal.

Think spinach leaves, cucumbers, tomatoes, lettuce, chicken breast, and maybe a handful of grapes or berries. The goal here is to eat a very filling meal to hold you off as long as possible. Eat as much spinach and lettuce as you want, with some cucumber, tomato and whatever other raw vegetables or leaves you would like to throw in the mix (stick to mostly green veggies and leaves).

Once you have been eating the high volume salad meal with the 4-hour intermittent fasting window for 2 weeks, it's time to open the window a little wider. This is where it may start to really get harder; this is where you will go to a 6-hour fasting window.

Which means if you wake up at 7am you won't eat until 1pm. Keep using all of the same techniques with water, coffee and tea. This is the stage in intermittent fasting where you must endure a little. Just like any form of eating, changing from the way you're eating and adapting to a new timing protocol does take a little bit of effort, as well as enduring the adaptation period. Once you are at a 6-hour window of intermittent fasting, you can either stop there or push onward to the 8-hour fast. I think both 6-hour and 8-hour windows can work great.

It really depends on your lifestyle; cubical desk warriors should be able to manage an 8-hour I.F. window, but hard labor workers will have a tough time adapting to 6. The benefit of fully adapting to the 6 to 8 hour window is the amount of calories you save throughout the day; this allows you to have a feast for your last meal.

Having a feast before bed really does the trick for making you feel full. Psychologically for most people, having one big feast is 10 times more filling than eating 6 small baby meals per day, or even 4 medium sized meals. You are able to eat more of what you want, plan to go out with your friends and eat whatever you want, and have the macros left over to do it.

I.F. provides you with the opportunity of a better lifestyle. Get lean or stay lean by eating just about everything you want. The less meals you eat, the more that one meal will fill you up both from a psychological standpoint and from a satiety standpoint.

It's not really about eating less - it's about being able to enjoy more of what you want later. Eating the majority of your calories later in the day will have you going to bed feeling satisfied with no cravings, and will even give you energy halfway through the next day.

I.F. + IIFYM for lean gaining and cutting.

Since I.F. is nothing more than a timing protocol for eating, it can be paired with any of the 3 eating/dieting protocols, IIFYM, I.E. or even meal plans. Although I wouldn't really see the purpose of pairing I.F. with a meal plan because of the nature of meals plans. The low eating frequency of intermittent fasting + IIFYM is actually my favorite method for getting lean or maintaining a lean physique for long periods of time.

I'm actually running I.F. + IIFYM to get into shape for the cover of this book. I like to call I.F. + IIFYM the dieting sweet spot because you still have total and complete control over your calories and macros, but you are able to have a large feast later in the day with almost whatever you want.

I am currently using macros 400C 65F 160P to lean down for the cover of this book. I started around 183 and will lean down to the mid to low 160's over a 3-4 month's period. At around the same time I am finished writing this book, and I should be entering the 160's. Here why I like this combination:

Why I.F. + IIFYM Works

It's the best way I have found to maintain a shredded physique for long periods of time while living a normal life. Since you're eating less frequently, you can have a much larger meal in the evening at home, or out with your friends. As long as your macros support it, you can basically go out and eat just about anything with your friends.

Take me and my current macros: if I eat only 75 of my 400 carbs before 6pm, then I have 325 carbs to play with for my dinner. Let's say I eat 25 grams of fat and have 35 left to play with, and I eat 100 grams of protein leaving 60 grams for me to play with. This means I now have 325C, 60P, 35F to play with for dinner.

Those numbers would make any flexible dieter happy at dinner. It does come at a price, though. Fasting 6-8 hours and then eating a high volume, micronutrient dense, high protein epic salad meal as the first big meal does take some getting used to.

One thing you really have to pay attention to is your fat intake; your fat intake is sneaky; it will creep up on you. Fat intake creeping can be a real issue with intuitive, that's why I like IIFYM a little better when it comes to staying really lean, or getting really lean.

Just a week ago I was not thinking about macros early in the morning. I had some coffee creamer with my coffee and a little too much coconut oil. What I didn't realize, was that the damn coffee creamer was low sugar, but to compensate these assholes raised the fat to 2 grams per serving! That's more than regular coffee creamers. I used 11 servings, shit dammit that's 22 grams of my life that just walked away from me.

Then the coconut oil, don't get me wrong coconut oil is my best friend from a health and performance standpoint, but damn does it pack a punch of fat. We are looking at almost 1 gram of fat per 1 single gram of coconut oil. I ate 28 grams of coconut oil for breakfast with my coffee. From an eating standpoint it seemed as though I was fasting. However, my fat intake tells us otherwise. Yep, I just consumed 50 grams of fat and didn't even realize that I just took out almost all of my fat while I am supposed to be intermittently fasting.

Let me tell you a secret - I always have my creamy coffee in the morning, fasting or not. I simply use coffee creamer that has 1 gram of fat and 1 carb per serving (15 milliliters is a serving) I try to stick to 6-8 servings with a large coffee and a couple tablespoons of stevia sweetener.

Pro tip: If you drink coffee in the morning and follow I.F., drink a liter of water pre-coffee, enjoy your coffee and then drink your second liter with water flavoring an hour or so later. Don't drink the coffee or the flavored water in a hurry. Sip it; if you don't keep your mouth busy it will get bored. As with any protocol, 5 out of 7 days you should stick to mostly a diet of only whole nutrient dense foods, but whenever you want to go out and enjoy a nice Italian dinner, using I.F. + IIFYM, you can pull it off and stay lean.

I recommend if you like Italian food, or any high fat foods, to plan to possibly drop a few carbs in favor of some fat if need be. I don't suggest doing this often, but once every week or two won't hurt your shreds, brah.

If you are maintaining a lean physique, your fat to

carb ratio matters slightly less, but when you're chasing the shreds, you need to watch it on the fat intake. For most of us, bringing the fat intake up to high will be a little harder for our bodies to deal with. Ironically, some people actually do better on high fat and low carbs, but for most of us, we do better on higher carb, lower fat.

When just following IIFYM with no meal timing, it can get irritating when you want something but you realize you screwed up earlier by spending your macros unwisely. With I.F. + IIFYM, you are always able to enjoy what you want later on in the day because you saved the macros.

I.F. + IIFYM is literally the complete and opposite from bro diet meal plans, so get ready to be under fire by the bro's - they will hate your guts and think you're the Anti-Christ.

Pro bodybuilders actually do have to eat constantly, because when your body is supercharged with GH, test, IFG-1 and tren, you're basically super human. But hey, I am natural and I preach staying natural, and if you're natural, food timing has much less relevance in terms of gains and getting lean.

For us natty lifters, it's all about playing it smart, working harder and smarter and staying consistent on our eating protocols. Using I.F. with IIFYM really teaches you how to budget your macros for when they will be most useful for you. Eating a big breakfast and then little baby meals all day sucks.

We want to be able to brag about the giant dinner we ate while staying shredded or getting shredded. We want to break this stupid dieting stigma of bland meal plans that make you want to drop dead before you do them.

I.F. + IIFYM is my personal favorite way to do things for photo shoots, contest prep and staying lean. Basically,

I won't go back to just IIFYM until I'm fully off season and not prepping for anything. I won't go full intuitive until I am in full bulk mode. This habitual method also works for many other physique builders. Give IFIIFYM a try!

5 Popular I.F. protocols

Let me first say that I don't promote any of these methods. In fact, a large part of section 3 is going to be dethroning popular fad diets and explaining why extremes are bad, and why there is no need for a crazy extreme diet.

1. **The Lean Gains Method** First of all, this means a fasting window of 14 hours for women, and a fasting window of 16 hours for men. Damn sexists, damn gender roles. I'm kidding if you didn't realize, women have much more fragile hormones than men. With that said, 14-16 hour fast, really?

   I am not saying that it's wrong, just that I don't really agree with it, or particularly see it helping any physique builders. During this fasting period, you consume no solid calories, only black coffee, diet soda, sugar free sweaters and sugar free gum. This method promotes fasting through the night.

   I don't like that idea at all. If we go to bed hungry, we won't sleep well and we'll be irritable and hungry; nobody wants to go to bed hungry. You can be flexible with this method, some IIFYM is permitted but not a lot. There is some alternating between gym days and non-gym days in terms of carb, fat and protein intake. While I am ok with a little carb cycling, cycling carbs, fat, and protein is a bit excessive in my opinion. No need for that hassle. I don't recommend this method.

2. **Eat Stop Eat Method** is even worse than team lean gains over there. This method uses 24 hour fasting. I don't even know why this is in the I.F. timing category. In my opinion, more than 16-20 hours is no longer I.F., it's just fasting, full on fasting. But hey you can still drink diet soda!

It's stated that resistance training is needed for this method to work efficiently. Here is the thing: if you do resistance training and use 24 hour fasting windows, you're asking for it my friend. This may work for .01 percent of people who aren't looking to build a physique, but if you're in it to win it, I don't suggest 24 hours of fasting followed by binging your soul out the next day.

I don't need to bring up scientific studies to tell you why this is bad. No counting calories, no weighing food, no restrictions. The method simply states to eat like a "grown-up" in moderation. This is a great method if you want to lose muscle mass on your fasting days and gain fat on your "eating" days.

My Spidey senses tell me this would create a nasty binge and purge eating disorder that would lead to a lower metabolism, muscle loss and higher body fat. While I don't believe in protein timing, I also don't believe that going an entire day without protein would allow you to recover from any workout. Methods like these may claim crazy results in short periods of time; what they don't talk about is how fucked you become, mentally and physically, in a short period of time.

3. **The Warrior Diet Method** is somewhere in

between lean gains and "eat stop eat." This method uses a 20 hour fasting window. The premise of this diet is to eat one epic meal, only one meal, a feast. I love the idea of eating a feast at night, but a 20 hour fasting window is going too far in my opinion. It's based off of eating in sync with the circadian rhythms. I do believe we were meant to eat 75% of our calories at night, just not all of them. I don't like extremes.

But hold on, this method boasts a big juicy contradiction. While you're supposed to be fasting, you are clear to eat a few servings of raw fruit or veggies, and even a little protein. While I think this is better than not eating at all, for 20 hours, we just defeated the purpose of fasting altogether.

4. **Fatloss Forever** is terrible. The only good thing is that it allows cheat meals. As you know, I don't like those 2 words because they imply that you're wronging yourself. Here's how it works: 36 hour fasts are followed by small windows of eating until you nearly explode.

Well, you're not supposed to eat that much, but ask yourself, what would a human do after starving themselves for 36 hours? You're supposed to eat sparingly on your eating days, "everyone loves full on cheat days," they say. Don't fast for 36 hour periods. For god's sake, you will lose all of your gains and probably screw up your hormones and be uncomfortably full on your "eating days."

5. **The Alternate Day Diet** is predicated off of eating very little one day, and eating normally the next day. Women eat 2,000 calories on their

normal days, and 400-500 on their "fasting days." Men go for around 2500 on normal days and still around 500 on their fasting days. They do actually have a calculator to show you how many calories you will need on normal and fasting days, which is generous. Meal replacement shakes are recommended on the fasting days, the next day you eat normal. The problem here is that this isn't even fasting, it's starve and purge.

Why These Are All Bad:

First of all, it kills me how most of the so called "intermittent fasting" protocols aren't really internment fasting. They're just using those words to market their starvation diets. I don't agree with 14-16 hour fasts, but when we're talking 20+ that's just not I.F. anymore at all. That's straight up fasting.

Almost all of these methods would ruin your relationship with food and turn you into a very unhappy person. We just have no need to fast in the 20th century. Maybe in hunter and gatherer times it happened, but we aren't hunter and gatherers anymore. We don't hunt, we go to the grocery store.

While I understand all of the philosophies used in these extreme fasting methods, none of them are the slightest bit practical. I suggest not to go over a 12-hour fast, and always to start your fast upon waking. Never start a fast mid-day and fast through the night. Fasting through the night is a recipe for disaster.

The Psychology of I.F.

From a psychological standpoint, I.F is very interesting. If you tell someone you're intermittent fasting they first normally wonder what "intermittent" is. Once you explain it to them, 95% percent of the time they tell you "I couldn't do that." I can't skip meals, they say, I would lose all my gains, they say.

There is this funny thing that happens where when you tell someone you made a change in your life and they perceive it as radical (a big change) that requires some effort. People often begin spouting out the rationale behind why they couldn't implement these same changes. Even if they wanted to, their body/mind wouldn't let them, they're just not build that way, and they wish they could. I have heard this all too much. Ironically, most of the people that try I.F. and do it correctly, love it. Here are all the reasons that I.F works.

1. You become much less food focused when you're just eating a couple of meals, post I.F. window. You don't think about food until halfway through the day. You are able to completely focus on your day without any worry of needing to take a break and stuff your face. Instead your break from work can have you relaxing. Since you have more time to get things done, most people typically become much more productive while running I.F.

2. Eating less during the earlier part of the day can help make you sharper and allow you to focus more on work. This may help you to get into the flow much more easily, as opposed to eating a huge breakfast and wanting to fall back asleep. For myself and many others, eating carbs in the

morning or just eating a lot of food in general leaves you feeling sleepy and foggy.

As crazy as it may sound, many writers actually fast while they're writing for the sole purpose of creative writing. For most of us writers and people that need to be mentally sharp for our jobs or careers, we have experienced a large increase in focus while running I.F.

It's my personal belief that just about anyone would be sharper and more productive earlier in the day from eating very little until mid-day. If you are someone who works at a desk and gets sleepy a lot, give I.F. a try. You may find yourself much less sleepy and much more focused.

3. The longer you can hold off, the more macronutrients you can save for later in the day, and the more satiated you will feel at the end of the day. Think of your macronutrients like money. You only have so many of them to spend per day. I.F. forces you to learn how to save for later in terms of macros. The "saving for later" mentality is a great mentality to have in life and in diet.

   When we save our macros for later, and we can go out and eat whatever we want with our friends, then have even a little macros saved over for a late night snack, it is so satisfying. There is nothing more satisfying than running I.F., getting to 6pm or even 8pm, and realizing you can now eat a feast and go to bed 100% satisfied.

4. Learning to have a mental budget of your macros is great because you learn how to save and invest.

If you saved most of your fat for the day and a lot of carbs, and were able to have a large steak dinner with mashed potatoes and red wine with a small dessert, wouldn't you feel good?

When you successfully save your macros and are able to eat exactly what you want later in the evening, it doesn't even feel like you're dieting. It's almost as if you can lose weight without feeling like you're on calorie restriction. Just last night I saved 245 carbs, 35 fat and about 30-50 grams of protein until 8:30pm. Literally, I had that much food left to eat. Since I'd eaten high volume, low calorie foods all day and drank 1.5 gallons of flavored water plus green tea, I was hardly hungry at all. What I ended up doing is making a double cookie melted dessert. I used one cookie from Jersey Mikes, one Snickerdoodle complete cookie, 2 servings of fat free whip crème, 1 serving of sugar free chocolate syrup, .5 serving of sugar free breakfast syrup, and made a masterpiece of a macro friendly dessert. I was happily satisfied afterwards.

The funny thing is that I still had a lot of food left to eat, over 100 carbs left, a little protein, and a little fat. What I decided to do was finish off my day with 2 servings of raisin bran and 360ML of 2% milk. After all that, I still came in almost 45 under on my carbs, 4 under on my protein, and 8 under on my fat. My targets where 65F, 400C, 160P, I hit 57F, 355C, 156P.

Anyone can do this with any set of macros. Saving them for later allows you to build basically whatever you want to eat, granted you have to fit it in. I could have finished my macros, but when you're on a cut and get extremely full, why keep eating if you're not hungry that particular day?

I personally believe that I.F. + IIFYM is the most powerful plan to follow, period, when it comes to staying lean for long periods of time. It's also great for your relationship to food. While you are counting macros, you're only really opening your phone to enter macros for 10 minutes out of your day, since you're only eating a couple meals. You get the control of IIFYM and close to the ease of intuitive eating. With all of this said, remember: a 6-8 hour fasting window tends to be the sweet spot for most people; some people do better on 4-5 and others 9-10, but for most people 6-8 works best.

Intermittent Fasting – The Bottom Line

Here's the thing, I.F. isn't anything special regarding fat loss or muscle gain. By now, hopefully you understand that. I.F. is a timing protocol that allows you to save the bulk of your calories for later in your day. It has been a crucial part of my own success in getting shredded year after year, as well as that of countless others. It tends to sharpen one's thinking, strengthen one's focus, and most importantly, it drastically increases one's satiety at the end of the day.

The biggest factor to one staying on a diet is the feeling of satiety at the end of the day plus achieving weigh in goals in a reasonable period of time. I sometimes can hardly even finish my food late at night because I have so many macros left to play with. At the same token, if I eat the same exact macros spread across 6 meals throughout the day, I am typically hungry at night. Being hungry at night either leads us to ultimately binging the night the diet ends, or binging before the diet is over.

The great thing is, if you drink flavored water, green tea and coffee while you're fasting, it basically keeps you 90% full until you actually eat. Now, granted once you get leaner than your body is used to, it will get harder and you will be hungrier, more often. There is absolutely nothing you can do not to be a little hungry and food focused when you begin to get shredded. But eating big, high volume meals with something satisfying before bed certainly makes it much easier.

When it really comes down to it, eating 6 meals a day or running I.F. and eating 2 big meals a day is a personal decision. Some people are just so habitually used to eating frequently that I.F. mindfucks them to the point where they get headaches, become irritable and turn into dreadful people. My theory is that they have these issues because they pre planned having these issues, so that they could give up after 3 days and scrutinize I.F. by preaching about how nobody should do it.

This is why I say that I.F. is mainly psychological; people either take really well to it and it works, period or they can't stand the idea and don't take to it whatsoever. I think I.F. is a great protocol fitted with IIFYM or intuitive eating.

It could work with just about anyone from competitive natural bodybuilders, to the overweight person looking to lose 100 pounds.

Breaking the Fad Diet Mentality

Fad diets are nothing more than food restrictive eating protocols with set calorie restrictions or calorie restriction calculators. They typically also come with an eating timing protocol, although you could run any slew of timing protocols with the diet. To be completely honest, you could run any timing protocol with any eating method; I.E., IIFYM, or a meal plan.

Fad diets are really nothing more than templates with highly marketed diet philosophies. I have respect for all of them because every single one of them can work, but none of them are going to give you superman results. It really depends on your own personal philosophy on dieting and food, what you should eat, what you're meant to eat, eating culture, etc.

Let's look at some of the top fad diets and break them down. Consider this: these different "fad diets" are at their core, simply templates. They are in a sense, a menu and structure to follow based off a culture and philosophy.

1. **The Mediterranean Diet** puts an emphasis on foods with healthy fats. Foods containing omega-3 fatty acids and other foods that support a heart healthy diet are part of the medi diet. This diet is rich in fruits, vegetables, whole grains, seafood, nuts and legumes, and olive oil. Sounds a little bit like the bro diet, just with more variety. The medi diet tends to be low in red meat and use of dairy products.

   The diet also recommends red wine in moderation. All in all, this would be a very healthy diet template to follow for great health. I think one of the reasons the medi diet is such a great diet is because it wasn't created for the purpose of marketing something. The medi diet wasn't created for weight loss or heart health, in fact it wasn't created on purpose at all.

The medi diet is the product of the natural evolution in the food culture of the people who live in the 16 countries surrounding the Mediterranean Sea, such as Greece and Italy. The medi diet offers a pretty wide variety of foods like veggie pizza, cooked veggie and rice dishes, beans, whole grain rolls or flatbread, grilled or steamed seafood, spinach leaves, salad with oil and vinegar dressing, as well as fresh fruits.

The medi diet is on line with most of my diet philosophy; it's highly nutrient dense and full of delicious whole foods, high quality protein, complex carbs, fibrous carbs and high quality fats. This makes it very heart healthy - a diet I could almost recommend.

Any diet high in great quality fats will obviously have a slew of amazing health benefits. If you've forgotten how important fats are in the diet, go back to section one and take another look at all the different powerful fatty acids out there that have the ability to do almost supernatural things to the body.

With all of that said, it means the medi diet is a fighter of cancer, Alzheimer's disease, Parkinson's disease and heart disease. The only problem I see with it is a lack of calcium, and I believe that with every diet you should be able to enjoy some processed food when you want it, just stick to 80-90% unprocessed whole foods.

This diet template could be used to make meal plans, eat intuitively, or even count macros. You have your 3 big ways of dieting (IIFYM, I.E., Meal Plan) and you also have your 3 ways of meal timing (timed, every 3 hours timed, and Intermittent Fasting), and the food variety you choose is the third decision. You could either A, study a diet like the medi diet; go "bro"; or C - Yolo, like most of us, which is eating whatever you want while hitting your macros and micros.

2. **The New Atkins Diet** is better than the old one. However, it still uses the same principles as the old one. The Atkins diet restricts carbs and emphasizes protein and fats. The entire premise of the Atkins diet is to cut back on carbs, the body's main source of fuel, in order to force your body to burn its fat stores.

On day one, to jump start the fat loss you will limit carbs to 20 grams per day. This can last anywhere from 2 weeks to two months. Once that first phase of the diet is done, you gradually up your carbs (it's basically a very slow refeed). Every week you will up your carbs about 5 grams; so 25 grams one week, 30 the next, 35 the next, etc. You slowly work up to 100 carbs.

The premise behind this plan is to maintain your new body eating 100 carbs a day for the rest of your life. I've never been a big fan of Atkins; I don't see the point in eliminating carbs. Ironically, fat has a lower thermic effect than carbs, which means if your calories were spread across fat, protein, and carbs, it would amount to more weight loss than just fat and protein.

Protein has the highest thermic effect of all 3 macronutrients - literally about 30% of the protein you eat is burned off as heat, and protein is also very filling. The reason Atkins works is because it's high protein and very restrictive.

The thing is, eating too much protein can be unhealthy. It's too much of a burden on your organs, not good for digestion, not good for PH levels. If you want to eat only fat and protein, opt for a ketogenic diet. I think the Ketogenic diet is much more well-rounded than the Atkins diet.

We just can't claim that favoring one macronutrient over the other is beneficial for weight loss, building muscle or general health. For 95% of people, I always recommend consuming fat, carb, and protein over just fat & protein. Just dropping to 20 carbs per day can actually be very dangerous for some people. Especially with women; a women's metabolism will take a dive 5 times quicker than a man's. This can eventually correlate to suppression of important hormones. Female or male, dropping your calories from whatever you're currently eating to 20 carbs per day overnight is never good.

3. **The Zone Diet** is based on resetting your metabolism. LET ME TELL YOU SOMETHING! Your metabolism isn't a fucking light switch. One doesn't just wake up one day, start eating whole foods and miraculously "reset their metabolism."

Yes, going from processed food to whole food and getting a better balance of macronutrients will yield a higher thermic effect on the food you're eating. But it isn't going to completely rebuild your metabolism.

Building your metabolism is done at the gym, with weights. Building more muscle, having a higher muscle to fat ratio, increasing your muscle mass and nutrient partitioning - *that* will increase your metabolism.

Other than the metabolism statement however, the zone diet is not too bad. It recommends eating 30% of your calories from protein, 30% from fat, and 40% from carbs. The only problem with this is that most likely your protein will be way too low. Always stick to .8-1.2 grams of protein per pound of bodyweight.

The types of carbs favored in the diet are beans, fruit, whole grains and veggies. That is great; these are the type of the carbs you need, props to the diet for getting that right.

Here's where my biggest issue lies: the whole balanced meal thing is just dumb and irrelevant. While balancing out your macronutrients on a daily basis is important, balancing them out equally in equally spaced meals is pointless.

The philosophy is that one meal should include a small amount of protein, a small amount of fat (like low-fat cheese or something), some veggies, and a piece of fruit. Now, while this sounds like a good meal, one I would personally enjoy, it isn't going to miraculously boost your metabolic rate. It doesn't align the stars for the perfect insulin level that will put you in some sort of mythical fat burning zone.

You want to know what will put you in a fat burning zone? Are you ready for this one? Sure you're ready? Alright, here I go! Be in a caloric deficit, BOOM! The food choices, the ease of use, and even the structure of the zone diet is great, and I have no problem with it, it could get people results.

I don't see it as being maintainable long-term, that 30, 30, 40 shit won't work for everyone and like 90% of these fads diets, you are skipping out on lots of nutrients since you will be cutting out some food groups.

One thing that is very bad about it is that most people who follow the zone diet will be on less than 1200 calories per day. That pretty much allows the diet to only work for a select demographic which is small women.

Two things that all of these fad diets have in common is that they're restrictive on food choices and they all put you on way too high of a calorie deficit out of the gate. You would lose weight on the zone diet, but not because you're in "the zone," but because you're hardly eating any food.

4. **The South Beach Diet** is based on the elimination of refined carbohydrates. Sounds like every diet plan ever, basically. People following the South Beach diet are prompted to focus on lean protein,

low-fat dairy, and good carbs – whole grains, veggies, and fruit.

You are gifted with 3 meals, one dessert, and 2 snacks - basically 6 meals. This seems to me like a variation of the bro diet. It's like bro + Atkins, but even better. You start out on super low carbs, only veggies and legumes, good fats, and high quality proteins, no fruits or grains yet. This is to get your weight loss jumpstarted.

I am seeing a pattern amongst fads; we always have some sort of jumpstart with these diets, which all use phases. Phase one can last anywhere from a couple weeks to a couple months, with the goal being to completely eliminate the processed foods out of your soul and lose a nice amount of weight.

Phase two adds in fruits and grains and continues the weight loss but at a slower rate. This phase lasts a while and should get you to your weight loss goal. Phase 3 is the forever phase; you simply add in a dessert and some healthy snacks and you're Gucci for the rest of your life. I like this a lot more than Atkins!

5. **The Military Diet** is a short term protocol designed to get 10 pounds off of very quickly for things like weddings and events, where you want to look "lighter."

The military diet was literally designed as a quick fix diet for people who need to fit into a wedding dress in the next two weeks, or who are about to go on a cruise, or for those expecting to see their exes at a party in the next two weeks.

Personally, I don't think you should scramble at the last minute to lose 10-20 pounds to bump into your ex or go on a cruise. And for god's sake, you need to do better planning for your wedding if you're two weeks out and needing to lose 20 pounds.

The whole premise of the military diet is to eat less than 1000 calories 3 days a week, and just 1500 calories for the other 4 days. Where this little fad diet is different is the food choices, the meals. For the first time, a fad diet allows processed food, it actually promotes it.

It's a breath of fresh air to see diet culture becoming less Nazi, but here's the problem: when you're fitting in processed food into your 1500 calorie off days, you're most likely putting yourself in a situation where you could become micronutrient deficient. There is hardly enough protein, so you would be losing a large percentage of muscle.

Here is a list of food items from the 4 days off – 3 ounces of meat, a small apple, 1 slice of toast, 1 whole egg, ½ banana, 1 cup of vanilla ice-cream, 5 crackers, 1 cup of cottage cheese, 2 hotdogs, 1 cup of broccoli, ½ cup carrots, 1 can of tuna. It seems to me like random processed foods and whole foods were just thrown together into a 1500 calorie diet.

Honestly, there are days when the things I eat can be a bit random, so I am not throwing a fit of hate on this diet, just stating what I observe. I couldn't find much on the 1000 calorie days;

I assume they are the same types of foods, just pushing more towards the whole food side.

The diet claims you will lose 10 pounds in a week. The diet also seems to be targeting small women. Here is the thing: if you're a small woman, you aren't losing 10 pounds of fat per week unless you stop eating completely + do cardio every day. If you're a small woman, you don't want to be losing more than 1 pound a week. To lose weight too fast as a woman is to risk affecting hormones negatively.

While I like the fact that fad diet culture is becoming less boring, it's still way too restrictive and feeds on our natural tendencies to want things as quickly as possible no matter how much it may screw us up. We want it quick; to look good for that moment to be remembered. Then when we get older, we love to talk about how good our bodies looked when we were younger.

Yep, you looked so good that one month you followed a starvation protocol and lost 20 pounds. You keep telling people how good you used to look, and we who have read this book will all know you're bullshit.

The things I dislike most about modern fad diet culture is the encouragement of the quick fix, the extreme weight loss idea.

People ask me all the time what diet I follow. If you tell the average person you follow intuitive eating or IIFYM, they will look at you like you're a drunk person. They expect you to tell them about the newest and greatest scientifically proven diet. But not you; you my friend are now in the loop.

The Worst of the Diet Industry

Want to have a little fun? Speed Round! Here are some diets that are 5 times worse than the first 5 I just mentioned.

1. **The Tapeworm Diet** is a real diet protocol. People purposely give themselves tape worms to lose weight. You inject tape worm eggs, then wait for those little guys to grow big and strong and eat your insides out, sounds like fun right?

2. **The Cotton Ball Diet** is an interesting one. Remember in section one where I mentioned that cotton technically was a carb? Cotton is mostly fiber, but a type of fiber that is indigestible by humans plus it has other things in its breakdown that are like poison to humans. Sadly, we aren't cows and we only have one stomach which isn't designed to digest cotton.

3. **The Sleeping Beauty Diet** is what old men give young women in their drinks at small bars. If you're asleep you're not eating, right? People literally and purposefully drug themselves to stay asleep for days on end so that they aren't eating. The problem is that you will burn muscle just as much as fat since you're not using them. This is the quickest way to end up dead or in the hospital.

4. **The hCG Diet** is sadly something I considered being a fat and depressed, unhappy 13-year-old. Luckily, I didn't go balls to the wall with hCG diet. I did drop that stuff on my tongue (just a

little pregnancy hormone called human chorionic gonadotropin, in case you were wondering), but it's ok because I did P90X at the same time. Anyways, the HCG diet is a 500 calorie a day diet where you *eat 500 calories a day!* Basically, the holocaust diet. You would die in less than a year if you kept that shit up.

5. **The Werewolf Diet** is just, I don't know what to, um, say. Hopefully, you at least become an alpha and can be part of Scott's pack on Teen Wolf. This diet is based on fasting according to the lunar calendar.

There are many other stupid diets which I will not burden you with, I'll just quickly say their names and be done with it: "Cookie Diet", "The 5 Bite Diet", "The Lemonade Diet", "The Baby Food Diet", "The Cabbage Soup Diet", "The Grapefruit Diet."

My Top 5 Fad Diets

Let's get one thing straight: I am not telling you to follow any fad diet, only that these make more sense than the previous 10 diet templates we reviewed.

1. **Paleo** is a diet based on foods that we hypothesize were the in the diets of early humans. Foods like meat, fish, vegetables and fruit, and excluding dairy or grain products as well as processed food.

   For the most part, this is how we should be eating 80% of the time, with the exception of dairy products. Diary isn't bad unless consumed in excess; the only people that need to worry about dairy are people with a lactose intolerance.

The paleo diet encourages a large egg omelet with peppers, mushrooms, and broccoli. You can also add diced turkey or chicken breast to the mix. This is a great choice for breakfast - high volume, high quality protein, highly nutrient dense, good fats, and nutrient dense carbs.

I am personally of the opinion that high volume, satiating foods are perfect for earlier on in the day because they keep you full and give you lots of energy.

The typical paleo lunch would be a large salad with greens, spinach, radishes, bell peppers, cucumbers, avocados, walnuts, almonds, and a little fruit. Chop up a chunk of meat and throw it in the salad. So far this is perfectly in line with the way I like to diet, and my whole dieting philosophy.

The only thing I do differently so far is put my first meal off for 4-6 hours. High volume tasty salad with tons of variety, that's a fantastic lunch. For dinner you can have broccoli, asparagus or roasted beets with your choice of grilled fish.

Fruit or dried fruit would be your post meal. One thing that really helps me take a liking to paleo is the 85/15 rule, 15% of the time you can eat things that aren't considered "paleo". Balance is always key in dieting; 100% methodology is never the way to go, and luckily the father of paleo understood this. You can't go wrong on the paleo diet. If you're looking for a template to follow with IIFYM, meal plans, or I.E., paleo is a great choice.

You can't really go wrong eating a high protein

diet, with high volume nutrient-dense carbs, and high quality sources of fat. The only criticism I have on paleo is that we don't live like ancient humans anymore, we aren't hunter gatherers and we also live a lot longer than our great, great, great, great, great grandparents.

The 85/15 rule excludes processed food and dairy. If only it didn't, paleo would be the perfect fad diet. Paleo has a lot of avid followers that get angry at anyone who dares to live by any other dieting template structure, which means it has really won the hearts of a lot of people, and there is good reason for that.

Eating this way is sure to make you much healthier than almost any other diet out there. Eating an 80/15 paleo/processed food & dairy diet would be a very powerful food template to follow. I have very few bad things bad to say about paleo; we just can't live exactly like ancient humans because we live in a much more advanced world today.

On the contrary, eating more towards the natural whole food side of the spectrum is exactly what we should be doing. I believe this diet started out its life being called the "caveman diet," and then became popularized as "the paleo diet." That name stuck, so just know if you hear "caveman diet," those two are the same thing.

Paleo and Mediterranean are very similar, the only huge difference is the paleo diet allows red meat, while the medi diet excludes red meat. The medi diet is a little low in protein for my liking but these are both great diet templates.

2. **Weight Watchers** or the original IIFYM? Weight watchers is a lot like IIFYM except it's predicated only on calories, not so much macros. WW is so much like IIFYM it's not even funny; you have a certain number of calories to hit every day, and you can eat what you want granted you eat mostly whole, nutrient dense foods.

Weight watchers has a whole dieting community; it's almost as if it's "the first of its kind". Out of IIFYM, meal plans and I.E., I would have to put WW in the IIFYM category; counting calories is counting macros.

It just almost deserves its own category because of its versatility and ability to adapt to almost any way of eating. On the contrary, I'm not huge on the points system. I would rather just count macros than use a points system to dictate my diet.

WW is great for anyone looking to get into shape, lose 100-300 pounds, be food conscious, etc. When it comes to us physique builders, it isn't ideal. We need to hit protein, fat and carb goals for the day, not just calories. Counting calories works for people looking to get a little fit or lose a lot of weight. A sharper focus is required for us physique builders.

All in all, I can't say anything terrible about weight watchers - it's a great program, a great diet structure, just not for extremists like us. The reason that we need to follow something bigger than a fad diet or a system is that we need to build our own system. Build our own meal plan, dial in our own macros, and learn how to eat intuitively. Fad diets and eating templates should be options and arts of study for us, but we shouldn't marry any one of them.

3. **The Volumetrics Diet** makes a lot of sense. It takes the principles of eating higher volume foods and exploits them. This is something that is proven to work, and is always part of my dieting methodology.

   We tend to eat the same sort of volume habitually, so if we up the volume and lower the calories, we lose weight. Since some foods are less energy dense than others, it means you can eat much less calories than you may be currently eating while eating more food.

   The fantastic thing is that these foods are typically much more nutrient-dense so you get a lot of bang for your buck when you use the methods of volumetrics. Literally a pound of low density carrots contains as many calories as an ounce of high density peanuts. Looking at and understanding which foods we can use to add volume to our meals, and using them strategically can make dieting on a caloric deficit almost painless.

   Using Volumetrics, 80/20, whole food to processed food, internment fasting and IIFYM is the exact protocol that I use time and time again to get absolutely shredded. Volume is one of the most important factors in a successful, long-term, healthy eating lifestyle, especially if you want to stay lean.

You could eat one pack of skittles and get the same calories you would receive from pounds and pounds and pounds of spinach. I'm not saying skittles are bad; what I am saying is that volume is very important when your macros start to get lower, when you have less actual calories and macros to play with.

If you're eating more than 20% high sugar, calorie dense foods, or high fat, calorie dense foods while on an aggressive cut, chances are you're going to cave and go way off your macros or meal plan.

I wouldn't exactly use volumetrics as a "diet plan" but as a major key to your success on IIFYM, or your meal plan, or even I.E.

I'm not going to lie - I have sabotaged a cut before by dropping my volume too low just for a day. That one day I got so hungry that my mind overpowered my logic and I went and binged, gaining 8 pounds of water weight overnight.

The volumetrics diet has very brilliantly laid out 4 categories of food; these categories are all relative to food volume.

Category 1 (very low-density) includes foods like low calorie fruits, vegetables, nonfat milk, and broth-based soup.

Category 2 (low-density) includes starchy fruits and veggies, grains, breakfast cereal, low-fat meat, legumes and low-fat mixed dishes, like chili and spaghetti.

Category 3 (medium-density) includes meat, cheese, pizza, French fries, salad dressing, bread, pretzels, ice cream, and cake.

And the Mack daddy, Category 4 (high-density) includes crackers, chips, chocolate candies, cookies, nuts, butter and oil. Oil is about the most calorically dense thing you could possibly consume. Your diet will major in C1 with and minor in C2, watch your portion sizes on C3, but don't restrict yourself completely, and keep C4 on the DL (down low for those that aren't cool enough to know what DL means).

This is the method that I use and the method I have used for countless clients. Long story short, it works. The way I use it is I stick to 75% C1, 25% C2 until about mid-day, in the evenings I'm leaning towards C2/C3, before bed I enjoy myself using purely C3, and occasionally I dip into C4 "in moderation."

Using this structure works great when losing weight. On top of that, water is the biggest volume tool of them all. I drink almost a gallon of flavored water before my first meal, so my hunger is blunted once I actually eat that first meal. I also drink at least a liter of fluids while eating. Always, always drink at least a liter of water while eating or you will not be satisfied.

4. **Keto Diet** is another diet that can be beneficial for some. Some people simply feel better and perform

better on fat as opposed to the body's normal source of fuel, carbohydrates.

The keto diet is known for being so low in carbs that your body is forced to adapt to ketones as its main fuel source. The goal of the keto diet is to put the body into ketosis. Ketosis is a natural process the body uses to help us survive when food intake is lower. During this state our body will produce ketones, which are produced from the breakdown of fats in the liver.

You won't actually be starving yourself, just forcing your body to use fat as its main source of fuel. The thing is, our bodies are very adaptive. When you take away carbs and overload your body with fats, you begin to burn ketones as your main source of energy.

A lot of people feel better running on ketones rather than glucose. I can't attest to it personally because I have never been able to bring myself to follow a keto diet.

To begin keto, you will be reducing your carbs to 15 or less per day. Obviously, you can't do literally zero carbs, because a little bit of vegetables and green leaves are needed. When following keto, you still have to get your fiber in and fiber is a carb.

The keto diet plays off of "net carbs" instead of carbs. What is a net carb? When you look at something like a cup of broccoli, you're looking at around 6 carbs; 2 grams of those carbs are fiber. Subtract the fiber from the 6 carbs and you will have 4 carbs left over, those 4 carbs would be your net carbs. Those are the carbs you use to meet your carb intake on keto.

Your total carb intake depends on your overall caloric intake; you should be eating 70% fat, 25% protein and 5% carbs. Now obviously the protein intake would change depending on if you were on a deficit or surplus, and your weight, age and gender.

The point is, you need to keep your macros at 5% carbs or less habitually to remain in a ketogenic state. If you observe spinach, it's so low in net carbs, you can eat a nice amount of it without bringing yourself out of ketosis. Spinach contains only .1 net carbs per ½ cup, lettuce is .2 per ½ cup, and cabbage is 1.1 per ½ cup.

Green beans, cauliflower and broccoli are a little higher in net carbs, but you should still be able to eat them. Here is a link to a great website for anyone looking to start keto; it even has a keto macro calculator, Ruled.me.

Like I said earlier, I have heard stories of people who don't react well to high carb diets who up and switched to keto, and all of a sudden they had tons of energy. I think keto has a lot to offer to anyone who doesn't particularly react well to high carb diets.

Some of us may feel sleepy and lethargic on high carb diets, some of us have issues with insulin, and some of us may just perform better on high fat.

I am not an expert on keto by any means, but I think it is a great option to try if it seems like you perform better when eating less carbs and more fat, or have more energy, or you have issues with blood sugar and insulin.

One thing I do want to get out of everyone's head is keto being this super special diet that will burn more fat than a fat/carb/protein diet. Keto doesn't have any profound fat burning or muscle building power; it doesn't put your body into any sort of super fat burning state because of low blood glucose levels and insulin.

Your body simply adapts to the new source of fuel you're giving it and uses it just as it would carbs. It's impossible to escape from thermodynamics.

5. **Vegan** is a way of eating that I am sure you are all familiar with. So, vegans are like extreme vegetarians. Not only do they not eat meat, fish or poultry, they also don't eat eggs, dairy products, honey or silk.

   It's as if anything is from any living animal or insect, they will not ingest it. I am not one to agree with extremist natures but that's a vegan for you. I am not going to go into the moral or ethical reasons behind veganism because frankly I want no part in it; that would be a completely separate book.

   The vegan diet has a variety of food choices like fruit, vegetables (obviously), leafy greens, whole grain products, nuts, seeds, and legumes.

   With all of that said, don't think for a second that you couldn't get fat following a vegan diet.

Vegan diets are some of the healthiest diets, especially considering dairy and meat products are harder on digestion. I would have to say that the vegan diet is one of the highest nutrient dense diet templates out there.

Since your diet is based off of leafy greens & fruits, your nutrient intake would be much higher than the average American diet by nature. The only really bug issue I see with veganism and bodybuilding is the lack of protein in the diet. It's very, very difficult to consume enough protein when animal products are out of the picture.

That even means no whey protein, no casein, no beef, chicken, egg, or fish. Almost every high BV protein source out there is associated with animals. Now, there are green foods, grains and legumes which are high in protein, but nothing compared to animal products.

That's not the only issue. Fiber is going to be so abundant on the vegan diet that just by trying to hit your protein goals you may be consequently injecting too much fiber.

The third issue is you have to eat a lot of vegan foods to hit decent protein goals which makes it very difficult to get enough protein when on a calorie deficit.

If you a vegan and a physique builder, I have one word for you "Tofu." Tofu is one of the only vegan foods that is high in protein, has a decent BV and doesn't also come with a ton of carbs and fiber per serving.

Tofu is about 6 grams of fat, 6.5 carbs, 2 grams of fiber, and 24 grams of protein per 150 grams. All in all, you can get your protein in on a vegan diet, but just know it will be much less practical, much more expensive, and a bit more technical.

There are a couple of other great vegan protein sources, but you really have to pay attention to your fiber. If your fiber gets too far over 1 gram per 100 calories you're going to tear up your stomach.

Too much fiber actually hurts nutrient absorption and can lead to loss of nutrients. The **80/20 Vegan diet** is something I'm much more a fan of. 80/20 in dieting is always better than any other number split.

I am not a big believer in 100% anything in terms of dieting. The 80/20 is like being a flexible vegan; if you want cheese pizza every once in a while, go for it. If you need whey protein (hint hint), go for it.

The vegan diet, with the option of a high BV protein source, would then be complete in my opinion. I love meat, but too much meat can be a bad thing. Our intestines aren't super-efficient at dealing with an overload of meat and dairy products. I believe that cutting them both down to a minimum is something that could be fun to try in an effort for cleaner energy, stronger workouts, and sharper focus.

I haven't personally tried this, but I do plan to in the future. Fitness isn't just about getting shredded, or being strong in the gym. It's about being strong in life.

Being more focused in your job or career, enjoying more energy, having stronger hormones, having fun, helping others do the same - that's what fitness is truly about.

I would never exile any dieting template; I think they are all worth a shot, all of the diet templates that make sense anyways. Vegan, Mediterranean, Paleo, Tropical, Keto, volumetrics are all powerful diets. Every single one of those diets has powerful methods and insights that we can adopt to use in our own diet. Let's open the dialect to the bigger picture of what dieting really is.

Poverty Macros are macros so low that you have to pay very close attention to your food volume, otherwise you will starve. Poverty macros are completely subjective from person to person.

For example, poverty macros occur for me when I get to about 250C 45F 160P. However, to obtain an absolutely shredded look for a bodybuilding competition or a physique photoshoot, I need to dip into poverty macros for a couple of weeks at times. Once I get to those macros or lower, things get difficult for me. In general, I have a tough time once my carbs go under 300g per day.

Everyone will hit poverty macros at different numbers because we are all different sizes, ages, genders, plus we all have different metabolic rates. This, everyone, is the point in your diet/prep where you start to get irritable; where every minute mishap of the day will make you angry.

You eat but hardly ever get full. When you're in this

phase of the diet, if you attempt to fit in highly calorically dense foods, you're practically committing diet suicide. When you're losing that last 10-12 pounds while getting shredded and drinking lots of flavored water, the taste of food, food volume, the size of your meals, satiation - it all becomes very, very important for your sanity.

One does not just make it through poverty macros without strategically eating super high volume. Here are the most important tips for servings through poverty macros.

1. **Water and Fluids**. If you drink less water than normal, the first time you will feel it almost immediately. When you're getting shredded, every craving, every bit of hunger, every irritation is a little more intense.

    The first thing to do is wake up and have a large coffee, or large green tea. For the coffee creamer, use a brand that offers sugar free, fat free creamer. I use Coffee Mate sugar free/fat free Italian sweet crème. This has been my creamer of choice for years. Seasonally, you may stumble upon some interesting fat free/sugar free coffee creamers. The more variety you can create with your fat free/ sugar free creamer selection, the easier it will be. Variety is very important for sanity when getting shredded on poverty macros.

    Use one tablespoon of stevia for sweetener. The amount of creamer you put in your coffee should be based off your macros. Since you're on poverty macros, I suggest staying under 6 servings of creamer.

    One trick I use to make more coffee and use less creamer, is simply to make the coffee weaker.

Put half the scoops of coffee you normally would in, then you can use twice as much coffee, and the creamer will have a much better sweet to bitter ratio in your coffee; volume is key here.

If you're using green tea, you can drink 2 large green teas with about 2 servings of fat free/sugar free creamer and a tablespoon of stevia. This makes for a pretty tasty tool of satiation to fight the emptiness of poverty macros.

You also need to find some sugar free flavored water staples. Personally, I use jolly rancher and Kool-Aid water flavoring. Green apple jolly rancher and watermelon together make a great tasting water. Get a gallon jug of water, use 2 water flavoring packets of your choice and a squirt of lemon juice. That gallon should last you though the day.

You have your giant flavored water, your teas and your coffee. If you take pre workout that is another little treat; if not White Monster drinks taste amazing and are great pre workout sugar free drinks, very tasty.

Just know this: when you're getting shredded, you feel everything much more intensely, you feel the weight more at the gym, you feel your emotions more, you get stressed easier, etc. Water is crucial to blunt these things.

2. **No Calorie-Dense Foods.** I know, I know, it's IIFYM and technically, you should be able to fit in processed foods. Here's the thing, you can still fit

in processed foods on poverty macros but they need to be low fat, low sugar versions.

If you attempt to fit in any high calorie foods on poverty macros, you will have no energy, be starving, and it will feel like you're hardly eating at all. Not only that, your workouts will suffer as well, killing your workout to fit in doughnuts will ultimately equate to you losing muscle because your volume in the gym is lower.

If you lose muscle, then your metabolism begins to slow down. If your metabolism begins to slow down, you will stop losing weight on your cut.

So not paying close attention to your volume while on poverty macros leads you to a world of shit. Metabolic rate slows, you lose muscle, fat loss slows, fun stuff. How do I know this? I have personally endured these mistakes for you guys, now you can learn from my fuck ups.

3. **Salad & Veggies are Life.** I am not kidding. Besides water, leaves, lettuces and assorted veggies are your biggest assets to your poverty macros. Spinach leaves are literally one of lowest calorically dense things you could possibly eat.

Spinach and romaine lettuce, and lots of flavored water will become go to buys when on poverty macros. They're highly nutrient dense, hold a good bit of water, and are very filling. This is why I preach your first meal of the day being a huge salad.

You drink flavored water, coffee and tea while fasting, then when your fasting window is over, that large salad will keep you full for a good portion of the day.

Here is a list of foods you can use to add volume to your salad: Watercress leaves, torn arugula leaves, chopped red onions, cucumbers, tomatoes, garlic cloves, romaine lettuce, bok choy, kale, chopped red peppers, radish, mixed salad greens, celery, chili peppers, cilantro, carrots, green beans, snap peas, green bell peppers, parsley, basil, salsa, mushrooms, sliced squash and zucchini.

Hopefully, you get the point. Those are all low calories foods that you could go crazy on in terms of volume. You could also add in veggies like broccoli, cauliflower and even assorted veggies. Building a salad with these foods as a base makes for a wide variety to build each salad, as well as creating a salad that is really colorful and tasty.

As odd as it sounds, the more brightly colored foods in your meal, the more satiating it will be, it's psychological but it works.

4. **Egg White Omelets**. Egg whites are a great high protein source and the perfect template for a super high volume meal. You can buy egg whites in a jug. Or buy the whole eggs and separate the whites from the yolks by tossing the yolks and whites back and forth in the shells while letting the white drop into the pan.

Buying a jug of egg whites is much more convenient but also a lot pricier. High volume egg white omelets are great high volume first meals.

This can be a great option to diversify your meals when on low macros.

Literally all of those same ingredients I listed for a salad can also be cooked in with your omelet. You can also find fat free cheese at the grocery store or supermarket, it's basically protein cheese. Yes, protein cheese is a thing, you're welcome.

Here's *my personal egg white creation* that makes me really happy. Keep in mind this is based around my protein goals. 10 egg whites, 2 slices of fat free cheese, about 50 grams of sliced tomato, about 50 grams of slices red pepper, 25-30 grams of sliced bell pepper, 30-50 grams of spinach leaves, a handful of mushrooms (30-50 grams), and sometimes I also add 100 grams of sliced cucumber or squash. I top that off with either some low calorie hot sauce like Sriracha, Cholula, Franks Red Hot or even occasionally, Texas Pete or Chipotle sauce.

Sometimes I use sugar free ketchup, as crazy as this may sound, you can hardly tell the difference between full sugar ketchup and sugar free ketchup.

With all of that, you have one delicious and filling omelet; add to that a nice low cream coffee or tea with a small bowl of berries, about 100 grams or so with fat free/sugar free Hershey's chocolate syrup, and you have yourself one satiating, colorful, tasty, poverty macro meal.

The goal with these poverty meals is to keep the fats to a minimum (under 10 grams, even under

8 grams if possible), keep carbs under 50 (under 35 if possible), and have the majority of your meal be protein.

Eating like this, saving carbs and fat for later in the day, allows you to enjoy yourself later in the evening. Having more enjoyable foods to eat in the evening really helps keep you satiated.

It's difficult to get any sleep when hungry. You could even have an egg white omelet with a salad on the side if you're really feeling like binging on volume.

You shouldn't binge on volume all of the time because it will eventually create an unhealthy relationship with food where you're obsessive about creating super high volume meals. But a meal where you're eating pounds of food can be helpful every once in a while. As your macros drop and you get hungrier and hungrier, your food volume must rise to the occasion.

5. **Strawberries** are much lower in carbs & sugar than most other fruits. Apples, pineapples, grapes, raisins, plumbs and especially bananas are all fruits you want to keep at a minimum when cutting on poverty macros because they are calorically dense fruits.

Strawberries are much less calorically dense than those fruits and are also packed with vitamins and antioxidants.

For comparison's sake, let's compare strawberries in grams to high calorie fruits. 300 grams of strawberries is about 24 carbs, 100 calories. 300 grams of raspberries is about 36 carbs, blueberries are about 44 carbs for 300 grams; apples are 43 carbs, grapes are about 54 carbs, pineapples are 39C, raisins are over 200C, and bananas are about 69C.

Get the point? Knowing which fruits are low and high calorie is very beneficial for your poverty macro longevity. Well, hopefully you aren't on poverty macros long, but at least it's helpful to know while you are on poverty macros.

Honeydew, watermelon and grapefruit are also great low calorie fruit options. Honeydew = 27C per 300G, watermelon is about 24C per 300G, and grapefruit is about 33C per 300G. Strawberries, watermelon, and honeydew are the perfect salad additives. 100 grams of strawberry, 100 grams of watermelon and 100 grams of honeydew are perfect fruit additives for your first meal/high volume salad. They are also perfect side dishes for an egg omelet meal.

6. **Save it for Dinner**. After you have had your large egg white meal & salad, dinner should be fun. Dinner should be a large quantity of meat with some complex carbs.

You have eaten super high volume all day for the sake of poverty macros, now is your time to have a nice meat and potato meal, literally. Stick to lean chicken breast, lean beef, filet steak and fish, or tofu if that's what you're into.

300 grams of sweet potato is about 60 carbs, 300 grams of red potato is about 48 carbs (if you

need to stay conservative or want to save macros for dessert), pick your weapon of choice.

You could also make mashed potatoes. You can find low calorie cream bases if you look hard enough. You can use low calorie almond or soy milk for volume adders, melt some fat free protein cheese on top for happiness.

You can add parsley, basil, salad, pepper and zero calorie butter spray to top the potatoes. (This is making my mouth water as I write, I do it for you.)

You can also make mashed sweet potatoes, they're surprisingly good, also baked French fries or sweet potato fries. You can use the same seasoning as mentioned for the mashed potatoes.

There are other choices other than potatoes for a complex carb, but not many other choices can be as tasty, fun, creative and filling for a dinner complex carb.

Rice can also be fun, you can season it about the same way, even add the cheese, but in my opinion potato is a bit more satisfying. Add some veggies to your meal like broccoli, squash, zucchini, cauliflower, have fun with it, and season them well.

This meal should be an experience. One of the biggest tips I can make to help you follow low macros is to enjoy your meals, enjoy the process of cooking them, find the right amount and type of seasoning that vibe with you, and realize that you really are doing a great job.

Pick your meat source, flavor that shit and saver the flavor of a tasty dinner. Dinner should always be the center of the meal day. I believe taking the fun out of dinner is not something you should ever do whether on macros or a meal plan. Dinner must be enjoyed, especially when you only have 200 carbs for the day.

7. **Protein Creations** will help you enjoy your diet, hit your protein, and save fat and carbs at the same time. Have you ever discovered making protein creations? What do I mean by protein creation? I literally mean creating brownies, pancakes, and sludge out of whey or casein protein powder.

   That's right, you can have your brownie and eat it too. Eating protein creations really helps up the fun when on low macros, but be sure to find a protein powder that isn't super high in fat.

   One whole egg + 1 scoop of chocolate protein powder + 2 servings of fat free whip cream + 1 servings of fat free/sugar free chocolate syrup + .25 to half a serving of sugar free breakfast syrup, and you have yourself a protein brownie, muffin, or pancake.

   Put all of those ingredients in a bowl, stir for about 1 minute, then decide what you want to make. If you want to make a protein brownie you're done, stick it in the microwave for about 1 minute to 90 seconds and you have yourself a protein brownie.

   Once it's done, you can put one serving of fat free whip cream on top, one serving of fat free/sugar free Hershey's chocolate syrup, 15ml of sugar free breakfast syrup, and if you have the macros left, 1 servings of low sugar fat free ice-cream.

You can find fat free ice-cream in just about every brand if you look hard enough, I use Breyers Vanilla fat free ice-cream. Breyers also makes strawberry and chocolate in fat free.

It's harder to find but if you venture over to Blue Bunny, there are some pretty spectacular fat free flavors. Blue Bunny has brownie sundae, mint fudge swirl, and caramel toffee crunch, all fat free and just waiting to top your brownie.

The point is, you can find some pretty amazingly tasty desserts to build, even while on poverty macros. Another great brand is Edy's, with their fat free vanilla chocolate swirl. One more honorable mention would have to be Skinny Cow; they make some awesome macro friendly ice-cream products.

Now you have a fully decked out protein brownie topped with all your hopes and dreams. Fireworks will explode in your poverty macro head as you eat this delicious protein dessert.

You can also add fruit to your brownie, either on top, mixed in or both. The size and amount of carbs will all depend on how much macros you have left for that meal.

If you want to make a protein pancake, you simply mix it the same way in a bowl and poor it onto a pan. Make sure the pan is pre heated with

Pam and your pancake should take less than 3 minutes to cook. Once the pancake is on the pan give the bottom side a bit to cook, then flip the pancake.

Pro tip - once you have flipped the pancake the first time, press your spatula against the pancake stretching the pancake out in surface area, this doubles the size of the pancake and allows it to get completely cooked. If you don't do this, you will have a smaller, fatter pancake with sludge in the middle.

You can also add fruit to your pancake, although I recommend adding minimal fruit to the mix as protein pancakes tend not to flip at all without breaking if you add to much density to them from fruit.

I tend to go a little crazy with the breakfast syrup since it is a pancake. You can find some seriously low calorie breakfast syrups, my top 2 are Cary's sugar free syrup and Walden Farm's sugar free syrup. Walden Farms has an assortment of amazing, practically calorie free condiments but you will be paying around $4 for a bottle of syrup or salad dressing, and it goes quick.

There is also an assortment of sugar free delicious toppings out there. Hershey's makes a sugar free strawberry syrup alongside their sugar free chocolate syrup.

Foaming at the mouth yet? Take a dive into Smucker's and you will find a sugar free hot fudge topping, and a sugar free Carmel topping. Even though it says "sugar free," it still has carbs, so you do need to use the toppings sparingly. The caramel topping, for example, is 24 carbs per one fluid ounce. You can use about ¼ to half a serving on your protein pancake or brownie.

Just about any tasty dessert item you can think of has a low fat/low sugar version, but a lot of times they're still pretty calorically dense so you do need to use them in moderation.

The other thing you can build is a protein muffin. This is simple mix of your protein ingredients in a coffee cup instead of a bowl; throw it in the microwave for 1 minute to 1 minute 15 seconds. When your coffee cup is ready to be taken out of the microwave, it will have a big fluffy muffin inside it.

Muffins can be great because you can fit a lot of fruit in them and since they're formed inside a coffee cup, their structure won't break.

For protein muffins, what I typically do once they're done is take them out of the coffee cup, put them on a white plate and then add toppings.

Fat free/sugar free Hershey's can be great toppings, but I like to save my going crazy on toppings, syrups and whip cream for my pancakes and brownies. I like to look at the protein muffin as a casual, tasty protein snack, and the brownie and pancake as protein desserts.

The possibilities are endless with protein desserts and protein snacks; you can build whatever the mind can conceive, and the great thing is that it's all trackable if you're counting macros, even poverty macros.

There is no reason for your diet to ever be boring. The protein pancake or brownie would be your post dinner dessert to finish off your macros. It's always helpful to eat something that satisfies you and makes you happy before bed.

The muffin is a great between salad and dinner meal to keep you full. At the end of the day, these protein creations are simply powerful tools to get you through your poverty macros.

So just to recap, the meal structure that works well for poverty macros goes like this.

Fast until 12:30 to 3 *using flavored water, coffee and tea.*

First Big Meal *will be a large salad or large egg white omelet with fruit on the side, or even a mix of both. (make sure to drink around a half a liter to 1 liter of water while eating this first meal.*

Mid-Day Snack *can be either a protein muffin, protein smoothie, or you can just fast and save your macros for dinner and dessert.*

Meat & Potato Dinner Meal *(make sure to drink around a half a liter of water while eating this meal)*

Before Bed Dessert *This meal should satisfy your soul, be it a protein brownie or protein pancake.*

8. **Low Calorie Condiments** are life. When dieting on poverty macros anyways.

- **Ketchup, BBQ Sauce, Mustard,** these are 3 of the most common condiments used to flavor chicken, streak, eggs & fish. Heinz makes a ketchup that is literally 1 carb per serving. Yes, only 1 carb per 17 grams. Normal ketchup is 5 carbs, so you could literally use 5 servings of this ketchup and it would be calorically equal to 1 serving of normal ketchup, all hail lord volume.

  Personally, I love ketchup on my eggs and sometimes fish & chicken. This stuff hardly tastes any different than full ketchup. Give it a try, just remember you will pay 50-75% more for this luxury condiment.

  If you want to get a ketchup that has less than a carb per serving, Walden Farms has you covered. For 3 times the cost of normal ketchup, are you willing to pay $5 for nearly limitless ketchup on your egg whites while keeping the carbs bellow 5 grams?

  Sugar free BBQ sauce is probably the most amazing and versatile low calorie condiment out there. It's a great salad additive, great on sandwiches, chicken, fish, steak, etc. Just know that you will hurt your pocketbook most likely with sugar free BBQ sauce.

  There are 3 really good, high quality brands of sugar free BBQ sauce that I know of, I have used 2 of them habitually myself. You have G Hughes smokehouse hickory, Walden Farms, and Paula Dean's sugar free BBQ sauce. They're all $5 or more per bottle no matter where you get them.

If you're looking for the best flavor, I would probably go with G Hughes. For the best price, PD. You can sometimes find PD in bulk at membership stores like Sam's for under $10 for a double pack.

If you are looking for absolute lowest carbs, it will always be Walden Farms. Both PD and G Hughes have around 2 grams of carbs per 30ml, while WF is over there with less than a carb per serving. I am a big Walden Farms buff when it comes to BBQ sauce. BBQ sauce can go quickly since it's so low in calories, you could use the whole bottle at a sitting in a salad and hardly touch any carbs. But don't, unless you want to spend $100 a month on sugar free BBQ sauce.

Oh, how nice it would be to be sponsored by Walden Farms, Arctic Zero and Monster. My suggestion is to use ketchup sometimes, hot sauce sometimes, mustard sometimes, and barbecue sauce sometimes.

There are a couple other brands of BBQ sauce that I haven't personally tried, like Simple Girl, the newest Walden Farms competitor, but at $10 a bottle they aren't going to be holding a candle to old Walden.

Luckily this book isn't about the sugar free BBQ sauce war, I digress. Walden Farms has a great tasting Honey Dijon for about $3.50 per bottle. At this price and this taste, you can't really beat that. If Walden Farms can get their prices down to $3 or even $2.88 a bottle, they would win my heart, and probably yours as well.

- **Sugar Free Syrup, James & Spreads** really do make life great. Let me start off by saying that there is an assortment of sugar free breakfast syrups, too many for me to go over. Instead, I want to go over my favorite choices, which are Cary's sugar free syrup and of course Walden Farms.

  Cary's comes in at $2.88 with about 6 carbs per 60ml, Walden Farms comes in at about $3.08 at less than 1 carb per serving. Now granted, Cary's destroys every other free breakfast syrup in terms of carbs per serving it, but it still gets demolished by Walden Farms since it's only an average of 20 cents more while having less than a carb per serving.

  They both taste pretty good, especially warmed up. You can use sugar free pancake syrup for just about anything. Just today I made a snack with a Baby Complete protein cookie, 1 serving of fat free Dryers vanilla ice-cream and 30ml of sugar free Cary's syrup.

  Absolutely amazing tasting snack with fantastic macros. The full macros for my meal were 4F, 52C, 10P. Something like this is a fantastic pre workout meal.

  If you wanted to opt more for a high protein meal, you could always have a protein muffin with 1 whole egg and 60ml of syrup. If you used Cary's syrup, you would wind up having a protein brownie with macros like 8-10F, 10-15C, 50-60P.

  We already touched on chocolate syrup but

my top picks on chocolate syrup are Hershey's sugar free and Walden Farms. Hershey's sugar free chocolate syrup has around 5 carbs per 32 grams. Hershey's sugar free strawberry syrup has about 4 carbs per 32 grams.

Walden Farms has chocolate syrup, strawberry syrup and caramel syrup, and they're all under 1 carb per serving. But you will spend $5 on these specialty items and you probably won't find them in stores; they will most likely need to be ordered.

Obviously there will be other brands depending on your particular super market. You could also look deep into the Internet thing and find some interesting stuff but these are my picks. They will best suit your poverty macros.

Chocolate and strawberry syrup can be nice taste adders to any dessert or snack, protein brownie, pancake, muffin, cookie or pizookie. One extra condiment that can be very helpful is I Can't Believe It's Not Butter spray. Spray it on everything for that extra little bit of flavor; it's great on protein creations, meat and potato meals, and dessert meals.

- **Hot Sauce, Salsa & Cream Sauces** can all be very helpful when using poverty macros. There are tons of hot sauces out there. There are some really strong advantages to using hot sauce as a flavor adder over other popular condiments.

  First of all, they're naturally low calorie; most popular hot sauces like Sriracha & Cholula are 1 carb per serving. To top that, they all have their own unique flavors to them.

Rest assured if you get some Franks Red Hot, Texas Pete, Sriracha and Cholula, you will have enough variety to keep things interesting without the need of any other sauces.

Another great thing about hot sauces is you will probably spend a 4th or less on hot sauce as compared to other flavor adding condiments because they cost less, and because they're so potent with flavor, you don't need to add as much.

Most hot sauces are around $2.88 to $5 a bottle, and that bottle will last you for 2 to 4 weeks most of the time. One of the best things about hot sauces is their versatility. You can put hot sauce on everything including eggs, chicken, beef, steak, fish, veggies, potatoes, rice, salad, etc.

There is always a large and diverse selection of top popular hot sauces at your super market, so you won't have to special order any of them directly. If you are cutting on a budget, then hot sauce will be your best friend.

Another powerful condiment to use in addition to hot sauce, or separately, is salsa. You have the ability to add a ton of volume to your salad and meat & potatoes meal using salsa. There are so many salsas out there that there is no reason to even go into that. Salsas are all pretty competitive in both price and macros.

Pro tip: go to a membership store like Sam's and purchase a jug of salsa instead of small containers at a smaller grocery store; you will save money doing so. Goyo & Pace Pico de Gallo salsas are great choices if you're new to the salsa game.

Another great option that you may not have thought of is fat free Alfredo and cheese pastes or sauces. Ragu makes a low calorie alfredo sauce that is really tasty with low macros. This stuff has 4 grams of fat, 2 carbs, and 2 grams of protein per ¼ cup of 61 grams.

For a cheese sauce, those are amazing macros. This is just like salsa and hot sauce in that it's very versatile; you can use parm sauce on just about anything - eggs, chicken, beef, fish, steak, veggies, rice, potatoes, salad.

One delicious meal you can create is a chopped parm chicken beef stew. You would add 1 to 2 servings of low calorie parm, add the chicken and beef to fit your protein macros, 1-3 cups of broccoli and 1 chopped red or russet potato. I recommend red potato to keep the overall carbs of the meal down.

All in all, you can create a very balanced low fat, macro friendly meal that you can customize to fit your macros. This is a great option for your "meat & potatoes" meal.

If you wanted to be creative you could take your hot sauce and mix it with your low cal Parm sauce to give your parm mix that spicy kick.

Yes, it's fucking amazing. With these 3 items you can literally turn your meat & potato meal into something you would see in a Mexican American restaurant, all while hitting your poverty macros and loving life.

- **Fat Free Salad Dressings** and low calorie salad dressings in general are very helpful to take a salad from bland to "salad of personality." I bet you didn't know salads could have personality, now did you?

The salad dressings I want to talk about are ranch dressing, thousand island, balsamic vinaigrette and apple cider vinegar. There are 2 main brands of fat free ranch dressing that I like to use, Hidden Valley and Kraft. Personally, between the two, I think Kraft has a much better flavor. Kraft is also much cheaper at just over $2 while Hidden Valley is well over $3.

With Hidden Valley, you get 6 carbs per 32 grams, with Kraft you're looking at 11 carbs per 34 grams, but it tastes much better.

As you probably know there is always the option to go with Walden and have less than one carb per 32 grams, but neither Walden nor HV can hold a candle to Kraft's taste in my opinion. If I were going to kill some carbs in my salad on occasion, this fat free ranch from Kraft would be worth the pull of my 11 carbs, even if my total carbs for the day were 200g.

Kraft also offers a fat free peppercorn ranch dressing, which is also on point. Remember variety and volume are your best friends when on poverty macros. When we take a look at thousand island, we are in the same boat, only we are between Kraft and Walden. Again, in my opinion Kraft is the winner here at just over $2 for the same 11 carbs, same great taste.

You always have the option to preserve carbs and get a container of Walden, which always comes in handy when you're in situations where you want to save your macros. Just keep in mind that it's about double the price of Kraft.

The best salad dressing, in my opinion, is fat free zesty Italian dressing because of the amount of flavor you get and it has about 1/3 the carbs of a fat free ranch or thousand island. Kraft makes an amazingly tasty fat free Italian dressing that I put on almost everything, especially salads.

It has about 3 carbs per 32 grams and only costs about $2. If you want to spend $5+ to get you some Walden Farms, well, be my guest.

Last but not least, vinaigrette dressings. Kraft has a lite balsamic vinaigrette dressing with 1 gram of fat and 4 carbs per 32 grams, and also a lite raspberry vinaigrette with 1 gram of fat and 5 carbs per 32 grams. Both of these products are around $2.

These are amazing choices to diversify your salads in order to keep your poverty macros interesting. Dousing your chicken and veggies in a vinaigrette dressing from time to time is also very delicious.

9. **"Make me a Samich,** but not just any samich, a "PM (poverty macro) samich". Well, what do I need to make you a PM samich, Lord Gainz? Ok, let me break this down for you Mrs. Queen Gainz. The first thing you will need is some Sara Lee bread, the "45-calorie" Sara Lee bread. It has 14 carbs, 1 gram of fat, 6 grams of protein and 5 grams of fiber per 2 slices. Pretty good stuff.

The only constructive criticism I have for Sara Lee is adding HFCS into the ingredients, when I don't believe it is needed. The good thing is that it only makes up a small portion of the carb intake of the Sara Lee 45 calorie bread. If not for that, this bread would be 100% perfecto.

The thing is, that's not enough HFCS to hurt you, granted you aren't making sandwiches every day. Stick to an egg white meal, or protein brownie for a snack most days, but if you need variety every once in a while, that's where this PM sandwich will come in to satisfy you.

Look at it like this: it would make a great weekend food item to switch up your snack meal if you choose to have that snack meal between your salad or egg white omelet meal and your meat and potatoes meal.

Second thing you will need is some fat free cheese squares. Both Kraft & Borden make great fat free cheese squares. The great thing about fat free cheese squares is that they have more protein so these cheese squares help you hit your protein while eliminating fat.

Kraft has 2 carbs and 4 grams of protein, while Borden has 3 carbs and 4 grams of protein. Fat free cheese never tends to be pricey; always around $2-3 for slices.

Fat free cheeses are another life saver because they become a protein source. We will go into that after we spell out how to build your PM sandwich. With just the Sarah Lee bread and 2 slices of cheese, you are already around 14 grams of protein!

Now it's time to pick your sandwich meat. There are tons of great brands so we won't go into that, but the important part is to pick a meat that has .5 or zero grams of fat per serving. Lean turkey breast is ideal; you can sometimes find it with almost zero fat.

Now all you need is some fat free mayo - Kraft has you covered. Kraft fat free mayo has .43 grams of fat per serving, 1.98 carbs, and .03 grams of protein, yes the label was that specific. It doesn't taste exactly the same as whole fat mayo, obviously, but it tastes pretty good, got to sacrifice to win, right babe?

All you need now is a slice of lettuce and a slice of tomato. You have just designed yourself a perfect PM sandwich for you to diversify with when egg omelets or protein creations don't tickle your fancy.

For 2oz of turkey meat, 2 slices of Sara Lee, 2 slices of fat free Kraft cheese, 1 Tbsp of fat free mayo, 100 grams of tomato and 50 grams of lettuce, you are looking at about 2F, 28C, 30P, not bad at all.

Obviously, you can play around with the turkey and cheese servings to lower or bring up your protein intake for the meal. The great thing is you won't affect your carb or fat intake too much by doing so.

Now that BAE knows how to fix you a PM samach, let's get cheesy. Do you know there is a fat free version of cheddar, mozzarella, cottage cheese and even feta cheese? Yes, fat free feta cheese is a thing.

I am not going to bore you with all of the nutrition facts of these cheeses for the sake of not being repetitive, but I will say that all of the fat free versions of cheese are also protein sources, which in my eyes is amazing.

Fat free cottage cheese is high protein, cheap and it provides a great additive to salads for upping their volume and protein. Cottage cheese is so high that you could use it as your soul source of protein on your salad meal.

Let me warn you of one thing before you consider going crazy on fat free cheese; it will make you gassy and very bloated if you eat it too much and too often. It can also cause digestive problems which sucks for multiple reasons. I have literally eaten so much cottage and feta cheese in a day before that my weigh in went up 4 pounds the next day.

You're just not meant to digest that much

cheese in a day. It will fuck up your digestion for multiple days if you over consume protein cheese. With that said, it's a great supplement food, variety adder, etc.

But you can't replace your meat and whey protein sources with fat free cheese. You can get fat free versions of shredded cheddar & mozzarella cheese at just about any supermarket. It's great for eggs and also salads.

We both know that feta is good on anything. Be like feta, feta is cool. If you don't have a dairy intolerance, you should be able to have fun with cheese and still easily get absolutely shredded.

10. **Oatmeal Creations and Poverty Macro Desserts** are the final pieces to the PM puzzle. I am not talking about your "bro dieter" bodybuilding, bland oatmeal. No, I am talking about oatmeal fit for Lord Gainz himself.

Ask yourself, would Lord Gainz eat boring meals of steal cut oats and a protein shake, or would he eat a tasty oatmeal creation of the Gods? There is no reason to hold yourself to a boring, bland life of boring oats when you can make those oats go to work for you as soul food.

Oatmeal shouldn't be looked upon as a boring bro food; oatmeal should be looked at as a template for making an amazing dessert meal to end your day of Poverty Macros.

Oatmeal creations can be great whether on poverty macros or not, but we know everything tastes so much better when on PM.

There are many different brands of oatmeal, but just for simplicity's sake, we are going to use the classic, Quaker. If you can find 50% reduced sugar Quaker instant oatmeal, we can get started! (p.s. the great thing about Quaker oatmeal is the amount of variety; there are a ton of different flavors, high fiber, gluten free, organic, whatever tickles your fancy, just thought you should know, I digress).

The best bang for your buck would be the 10 packs containing 4 packs of Maple Brown Sugar, 2 packs of Cinnamon Spice, and 4 packs of Apples & Cinnamon. You can get that 10 pack for under $3 which makes oatmeal great for poverty macros and macros on a budget.

Without further ado, here are the macros on these oatmeals: Maple Brown Sugar = 2F, 24C, 4P; Apple Cinnamon comes in at 2F, 22C, 3P; Cinnamon Spice comes in at 2F, 24C, 4P.

If you really want to get some low macro oatmeal and are willing to spend a little more, "Better Oats Fit Instant Oatmeal" makes a Maple BS with macros 2F, 18C, 3P. Their other flavors like Apple S, Cinnamon, etc. are all about the same macros, but expect to spend about $5 per 10 packets.

The most important items to buy to flavor your already tasty oatmeal are I Can't Believe It's Not Butter Spray, sugar free breakfast syrup, and sugar free chocolate syrup.

The 2 best fruits I recommend are blackberries

and raspberries for their low carb nature. Blackberries are about 10 carbs per 100 grams with one gram of protein; and Raspberries are about 12 carbs and 1 gram of protein per 100 grams.

Now, obviously strawberries fit into this low calorie fruit orgy, but you most likely already ate a ton of strawberries in your volume salad earlier, so we need to diversify. Besides, smaller berries fit in oatmeal better.

With 1 packet of Maple BS or one of the other 2 flavors, 30ML of sugar free breakfast syrup, 2-4 sprays of butter spray, 100 grams of blackberries and 100 grams of raspberries, you have made yourself a very tasty nighttime dessert. In total, you're looking at around 2F, 50C and 4P.

I recommend using Cary's or Walden Farm's syrup for this meal, just to keep the carbs down. You can also use Hershey's chocolate syrup in place of the breakfast syrup, or you could mix 8 grams of chocolate syrup and 15-20ml of breakfast syrup.

One of the greatest additives to your oatmeal is low calorie Greek yogurt. You drop the fruit, and use a very small amount of syrup in favor of some Greek yogurt. This is an excellent option if you need to hit some protein in this last meal.

There are a ton of choices for low fat and fat free Greek yogurt. The five kinds I use are Yoplait, Dannon, OIKOS, Dannon Light & Fit, and CHOBANI. They all have tons of great flavors. I wouldn't say that any of them are really superior to the others. They all have their own unique personalities. I just tend to get what's on sale or what I seem to be craving at the time.

I believe you should try all brands and all flavors, it makes dieting fun. Let's use CHOBANI as a tribute, although they are all very balanced and competitive in both price and macros. If you're looking to up your protein for the oatmeal, CHOBONI plain Greek yogurt has an amazing 0F, 11C, 22P. If you add that to your Maple BS oatmeal with 30ml of breakfast syrup mixed in, you are in for a very filling treat. Just for kicks, let's add 50 grams of raspberries and 50 grams of blackberries. In total we are looking at 2F, around 48-50C and around 29-30P.

Those are amazing macros for a super tasty before bed dessert. If you are looking to hit macros with more balanced carb to protein ratios, you can drop the fruit in favor of vanilla or any other flavored Greek yogurt. I will be using Vanilla CHOBANI for these macros.

One packet of Maple BS instant oatmeal, 1 cup of Vanilla Greek yogurt, 30ml of Cary's sugar free syrup, and 8g of Hershey's low calorie syrup = 2F, 43C, 16P. That last option works best if you still have a lot of carbs to play with but very little protein.

Greek yogurt is also a great topping to add to any protein muffin, brownie, or pancake for a snack meal or protein dessert. If you ever want to try something really tasty, try adding Greek yogurt to a Baby Complete Cookie; it will touch your soul while getting in 16-26 grams of protein depending on your choice of Greek yogurt.

You can also mix the oatmeal into your protein batter when cooking a protein creation. Then top off that protein creation with fat free ice-cream or Greek yogurt depending on your macro situation, with some sugar free syrup, BOOM!

One of the most classic things you can do is dump a scoop of whey protein onto your oatmeal fresh out of the microwave. This is what you do when you need to hit a hefty amount of protein before bed. If you have never mixed whey protein with oatmeal, I shall now abduct you into the clan of bodybuilders, we all do it.

Seriously, almost every single one of us has thought up the great idea of adding whey protein to our oatmeal, then we mixed it and felt very accomplished and satisfied with the result. If for some reason you have a ton of protein left to hit because you decided to eat a lot of carbs early in the day and did not pay attention to your protein intake, protein oatmeal is a great option to salvage your night dessert or a protein brownie, obviously.

Personally, I am a big user of the Walmart protein, chocolate peanut butter by Body Fortress. The odd thing is I almost never make protein shakes. In fact, I never recommend protein shakes when on a cut because I don't recommend drinking your calories when cutting; it's simply unsatisfying.

If I need to hit up some whey proteins at the

end of the day, I will mix 1 scoop of my cheap wally world protein with one serving of Maple BS, 30ml of Cary's breakfast syrup and a couple sprays of butter spray. This makes for a very tasty chocolate peanut butter protein oatmeal mix. Macros on this meal are 6.5F, 34C, 34P, practically the perfect protein/carb dessert before bed.

If you still have some macros left you can add some fruit or Greek yogurt to complement your protein oatmeal. Build your oatmeal dessert based off the macros you have left.

I have one more secret weapon for if you ever need a volume adder which is really tasty for a snack or late at night. What am I talking about? Sugar free JELLO or as I like to call it, "Protein JELLO."

You can find sugar free JELLO at just about any supermarket, especially Wal-Mart. Here is the awesome thing: one packet of sugar free JELLO is 1 gram of protein, no carbs, no fat. There are many brands of sugar free gelatin, it doesn't even have to be JELLO.

The amazing thing is that this is a great snack at any time of the day; a couple packets of this stuff will help you feel full, while hitting 2 grams of protein and it tastes great, especially when on poverty macros.

I am not going to lie; in my last contest prep I binged on sugar free JELLO sometimes. Seriously, I would eat 10 packets at a sitting. I don't suggest binging on anything, but occasionally it's nice to build a super high volume sugar free JELLO dessert.

One very tasty dessert you can build out of sugar free JELLO mix is fruit, chocolate and syrup JELLO mix. It's fairly easy to make, you first need to buy the JELLO powder. Get your JELLO stirred, heated and ready to put in the freezer. Before you put your JELLO in the freezer, add 200 grams of assorted blackberries, raspberries, 32 grams of sugar free Hershey's chocolate and 30ml of Cary's breakfast syrup or Walden Farms.

The macros will be different depending on the amount of JELLO you use, so I will leave that to you. This makes for a very tasty dessert which is super high volume with very low macros. We are looking at under 40 carbs, no fat, and 10-15 grams of protein depending on how much JELLO you use.

Poverty Macro Conclusion

I could never possibly list all of the foods and techniques used to make PM easier, but these are the most powerful foods and most valuable tips to follow. There are literally noodles that have almost 0 calories, ooh and diet soda is awesome when on PM. I am not saying to drink diet soda all the time, just that it can add personality to your diet a couple of days a week.

The point of this subchapter is to explain to you how to work your way around feeling like you're starving and thinking you can't do this, because you can. This stuff is only as hard as people make it. Learning how to cook and learning how to enjoy your food while eating less actual calories is very satisfying if you do it the right way.

If you are someone who likes to stay lean year-round, these same methods can be used to keep you from gaining too much weight on a lean bulk. These methods, foods and recipes can also work great while taking a more intuitive approach to dieting, or even meal plans.

Doing something as simple as switching your 2% milk for a 35 calorie almond milk would reduce your calories by a pretty large margin per week. Making small adjustments to your condiments, the way your flavor your food, your snacks, meal timing, etc. can completely change the way you think about dieting.

The entire reason I wrote this book at all was to both shed a light on what you don't have to do and also to explain to you how easy it is to actually follow a diet that will get you shredded; that will allow you to build a lot of muscle all while enjoying that diet very much. Learning how to work with macros on a PM scale will give you the tools and knowledge to stay lean all year, to look your best all of the time.

Think of it this way: when you have little money in your bank account but know how and where to budget it, where to allocate it and where to invest it, that educates you. You learn how to deal with it and be affected by it on a small scale, and allocate it to things of the highest leverage in order to get you to your financial goals.

It's the same way with macros and dieting. If you can learn how to feel satisfied, perform well and get somewhat full on 40F, 150C, 150P, you would be surprised how easy it will be to maintain 60F, 300C 150P on a lean bulk.

Bulking on a Budget

- Bulking on a budget is something we all have to do; learning to budget the money you spend on food while bulking is crucial. Believe it or not, you can actually get every food item you need to bulk up without killing your checking account.

  One other thing; try to justify fitness as "your business" in some way; you can use protein supplements, pre workout, protein cookies, and basically all "supplement food" that has to do with your "fitness career" as a tax write-off.

  All you really need to do for fitness to be your business is to think of a name, it can be your name plus 'fitness' or something like that. Everything I do falls under "Jordan Miller Success By Design." Once you have a name in mind, go to the court office and make it official; it's less than $20 and grants you the legitimate the power to use of any supplements as a tax write off.

  You can also write off your gym membership, gym clothes, gym accessories, etc., as long as you have an actual business. What I mean by this is, you are in some way helping others, even if it's just an Instagram page where you post pics and give advice.

  If you compete, or are ever thinking about competing, this is also a legitimate business endeavor because you spend a lot of money to get up on stage, shredded. The whole ordeal of contest prep involves money coming in and money going out, and some contests offer money prices and pro status, which is also a return for your business.

Long story short, if fitness is something you take seriously, and it betters you and you help others, it's your business. You can use the money you invest in fitness as a tax write off.

Let's get to the actual food items you need to survive (by the way you cannot write off actual food). You will need 1-2 staple carb sources, 1 staple fruit source, and one staple veggie source; you will also need 1-3 staple protein sources, one staple fat source, one staple condiment flavor adder, as well as cooking spray. Protein is always going to be the most expensive macronutrient to satisfy but remember, you only need .8-1.0 grams of protein per pound of bodyweight to make GAINZ when bulking.

Let's take a trip to Wal-Mart and do some calculations - you may be surprised to know that you can end up spending less than $200 a month total on bulking foods, but it's true, you can. Let's first look at staple carb sources; rice and oats are two great staple carb sources.

- You can get 2 5lb bags of great value white rice for about $5.50 or $2.25 a bag. That's about 53 servings of white rice, this should last you about a month. You can find 1 box of great value Maple BS oatmeal for $2.98, which contains 20 packets.

I suggest either 2 boxes of Maple BS or 1 box of Maple BS and 1 box of the variety mix. The variety pack has 4 blueberries & cream, 8 peaches

& cream, 4 bananas & cream and 4 strawberries & cream. This should do you for carbs. Yep, $11 for a whole month of carbs.

- The Birds Eye California Blend is the perfect veggie staple for the variety. The BEC blend comes with broccoli, carrots and cauliflower. You can get 2 bags for about $11 or one bag for $5.98. 2 bags should do you for about a month.

- You can get bananas for about .57 cents per pound, which makes it one of the best bulking carbs ever, and it also nicely fills the role of fruit. You are looking at basically 2 bananas per pound, so let's say you eat 2 a day, that's about $17 a month total for fruit, or $4.25 a week, not bad.

- You can get chicken breast at about $1.99 per pound. Chicken breast can be a bit pricey for a protein source, so we will only get a portion of our daily protein from chicken, about 8 ounces a day. That's 8 ounces of chicken per day, which is about $30 a month for chicken, this puts you at about 48 grams of protein for the day.

- You can get 1 dozen Sunny Meadow eggs for $1.24. Eating around 4 eggs a day will get you around 24 grams of protein and 20 grams of fat. This puts your protein at 72 grams per day. You're looking at around $12.50 a month for eggs.

- You can get Great Value canned tuna for about $2.72 per 4 pack, not bad. For 1 can of tuna a day you are looking at around $20 a month for tuna, which is about 7-8 4 packs. One can of tuna is

20 grams of protein which puts you at around 92 grams for the day.

- Let's not forget that rice, veggies, oatmeal and bananas also have a little protein. We'll estimate that from all of those food items together, our protein would be at around 102-105 for the day.

- You can get a jug of Body Fortress Whey Protein for about $17.98, or get 2 for $36. The whole jug has around 540 grams of protein, 1080 for two jugs, which is about 36 grams of protein per day. This puts your total at about 140 grams of protein for the day.

- For fats, 2 containers of Great Value peanut butter will do you for a month for about $3.06 or $1.53 per jar. This should get you around 16 grams of protein a day, 19 carbs a day, and 35 grams of fat per day, for a month.

- All we need now are a few condiments, I choose hot sauce and cooking spray. You can get Great Value hot sauce for about .88 cents, get 2 of them. This should last you about a month for $1.76. Pick up two 8oz bottles of Great Value butter flavored cooking spray for $3.06 or $1.53 per bottle.

That's all you need. Now that's bare minimum, but the point here was to show you how cheaply you can make out when need be. We are looking at around $145 a month total, just to be safe, let's round it up to $150. We will also add some tax and estimate that at around $162.

This is how tight you can budget when times are tough. We have all been there, or are currently there. You could easily up your carb variety, protein intake, and add another fat source in and still be under $200 per month easy.

The amount of money you spend will be in direct correlation to your gender, metabolism, bodyweight and lean body mass. Your 120lb woman could probably get by bulking on much less than $150; probably around $125 a month, while your 240lb male, 6 foot 4 bodybuilder with a fast metabolism is probably going to spend $300 a month on food, minimum.

What I have given you here is a template; the food prices will vary, the economy will vary, but these will always be your best bang for your buck food items when bulking on a budget.

One thing that will save you a little money is trying to get your calories from both a surplus of fat and carbs. You can bring your calories way up just by using peanut butter and eggs for extra fat, that plus your carb sources like oatmeal and rice will allow you to get a good amount of calories in at a lower cost.

Whenever you decide to cut down, just know that using any of the foods from poverty macros would be at the complete opposite end of the spectrum in terms of food cost. When going to poverty macros you will easily double or even triple your food expenditure per month.

Low calorie, and virtually calorie free versions of foods are double, triple and sometimes four times the price of the cheap, original versions.

I recommend building your metabolism up so that you can eat more when cutting by building muscle, and also using cardio to put yourself in a caloric deficit, plus out of gym physical activity. Then you will minimize the money you spend trying to get super low calorie PM food.

All in all guys, if there's a will, there's always a way to

make it work, to make it fit into your current lifestyle and your current financial situation. Minimizing the amount of money we spend on food and allocating it to the things that will help us grow in life financially will allow you to eat whatever you want, whenever you want in the future.

SECTION 4

THE PSYCHOLOGY OF FITNESS – LIVING THE LIFE

Why Most People Never Even Begin

The reason that most people fail at fitness is lifestyle. Building a physique, becoming strong, powerful, lean, and healthy is not an event. Becoming all of those things is a lifestyle.

Being in the fitness game for over 10 years, I have seen a lot. The most common thing I see as an online coach is people who aren't committed. Someone will reach out to me for advice, to look into one of my programs, to coach them, to build them a diet plan, but then never follow through.

This may sound like common sense, but there is no magical advice that creates massive success in building the body you want. There is no perfect program that will give you god like gains in a month; there is no secret diet plan that will turn you into a shredded natural bodybuilder.

Do you know why things are marketed as "the secret to ripped abs", "the secret to big biceps", "the secret to a big chest"? Things are marketed that way because society thinks that there are these profound secrets that we bodybuilders and powerlifters use to get shredded and make gains.

I have talked to so many people over time about taking their health and fitness more seriously that I can chat with someone for all of 1 minute and can tell by the tone in their voice if I will ever hear from them again. Most people need to be told they may die if they don't change their eating habits before they actually make a change.

Some people actually dig themselves into disabilities by eating shit all of the time, eating much more of it than their bodies can handle, all while being completely sedentary all day. The part of this situation that really bothers me is that these people are allowed to live on disability, which inspires even more laziness and bad eating.

Everyone has a breaking point; chances are if you're not passionate about getting fit, if you haven't reached a breaking point, if you haven't already decided what it's going to be, when, and why, then you're not going to do anything but keep sitting there feeling sorry for yourself.

Do you know what my breaking point was? I couldn't take being picked on anymore at age 12 and a half. I was

12 years old with man boobs; really short, great target to pick on. I was always addressed in middle school as "faggot".

Let me state for the record that I am straight - this was a word used in middle school as a weapon to discriminate against kids who were circles in a square school. I got into a lot of fights in middle school, some I lost, some I won. I was little and fat, 11 inch arms, 36-inch waist, 5 foot 3 inches tall, 28-30% body fat.

Girls made fun of me, guys shoved me, I even once had a soccer ball kicked in my face for no reason, then was called faggot, after which a small brawl began.

For whatever reason, I did more kicking than punching in that little 1-minute fight, yep I was an awkward fighter. Even though I sucked at fighting, the one thing about me was that I never backed down.

In 8th grade I was jumped, my right leg was completely snapped up and I was told I may never be able to walk right again, that I would never be able to bear a lot of weight on this leg or squat very deep. I was home bound for months playing Halo 3, eating hot Cheetos, and drinking game fuel. I had isolated myself and could not endure the thought of leaving my room.

I pondered, should I commit suicide? Literally, all I have is this Halo game; nobody else likes me and I am a burden on my mom and dad. My uncle, who I looked up to, had just passed away weeks ago. We had inherited all of his guns, and he had a lot of guns. Two 9mm's, 1 Glock .45, 2 shotguns, one long barrel, one short, 2 riffles, one SKS, and one .22 trainer gun.

He also had a .357 which was my personal favorite. Needless to say, I felt like shit after he died and I had my leg shattered. I had no self-worth, I felt soulless. There were several times where I came very close to suicide with knives and guns.

This is hard to say, so get ready to read it. There were multiple times where I had guns in my mouth with the firing pin cocked back, contemplating less than a millimeter of finger movement on the trigger of a weapon that could put me out of my misery.

That was my breaking point. Everyone has one. Long story short, I always had that 1% of my being that kept my finger from squeezing the trigger or slitting my throat. I decided that there had to be more to me than an empty shell.

At that precise moment I asked my dad to take me with him to the gym. The rest is history. That 1% of my heart and soul must have known that I had something greater inside me than darkness and emptiness. The fitness lifestyle has been a key element of my life ever since, it saved me.

Let me say this, whether you have a breaking point like that, or you just know deep down that you need to change, DO IT! You owe it to yourself to be something. I want to see you succeed and I want this book to have an impact on your life.

This can't just be another fitness book that you spend X amount of dollars on just to put it in the corner of your dusty book shelf. The first step is realizing that you do need to make some changes, the second step is deciding that you are going to make the change, the third step is the change.

10 Reasons

The single most prevalent reason that someone doesn't do something is not having enough fuel to do it, not having enough reasons. If all you have to go on is "I need to start working out," you never will. If your only reason to start dieting or eating better is "I need to be in better shape," you never will be.

If the reason for getting off your ass is, "I need to be less lazy," you never will. You need to have at least 10 compelling reasons to fuel you forward. I don't mean made up reasons that have no relevance. I mean 10 reasons that strike you to your core. 10 reasons that are of such importance that you're no longer pushing yourself to change, you're being pulled to change.

Start with 10 reasons, eventually you will develop 100's. By that time, you will never stop; you will change your life and continue to grow. Without further ado let me name 10 different types of reasons that can fuel your journey.

1. **"I want people to be sexually attracted to me, I want to be more sexed up."** Don't lie. We all have a want to be more sexually attractive in clothes and naked. Saying you're not doing it for that reason is like a business owner saying "I don't do it for the money."

   That may not be the center of our focus, but in the back of our minds we all went to be sexually attractive, confident and have money, it's in our nature. Contrary to popular belief, you don't just walk into the gym and start dieting and become that way.

   There are tons of shredded and built guys and

curvy women in the gym that just don't have it. You want to know what makes certain people in the gym confident and highly attractive? It's not how ripped they are, or the size of their booty or biceps - it's their determination to move forward.

The confidence you receive from setting and hitting goals every day on your diet, in the gym and in life is like no other feeling, money can't buy this feeling. The first week that you set goals and achieve all of them you will be hungry for more.

The more, small goals you set and achieve, the more powerful, confident, and sexually attractive you become. There is nothing more satisfying than hitting a 45-minute session of high intensity cardio and finishing every single minute of it, down to that last 5 seconds and turning off the cardio machine at exactly 45:00.

There is nothing more attractive than someone who sets goals with both diet and training and goes after all of them with fire, and achieves them. It's not the actual look that gives someone that attractive energy, it's the work, the days spent grinding, the months spent grinding, the years spent grinding.

Nobody can ever take that from you; that will completely change your life more than anything else. It's completely priceless to be able to look in the mirror and have respect for the person looking back at you. You know that person looking back at you gets shit done, makes things happen, and does everything he or she sets out to do.

You become more and more confident, take on bigger and bigger goals, the world seems to be yours, you cannot fail, success in inevitable. That person you have become? That person is incredibly attractive. The great thing is you won't need anyone to tell you it's attractive because *you* did it, *you* put in the work, and *you* became this mentally stronger and powerful human being that makes moves.

2. **"I want to look in the mirror and love what I see."** Self-hatred and low self-esteem are 2 nasty things that sedentary people who eat junk all day feel. If you don't, that's great, but for the people that do, this is one of the most powerful reasons you need to get into the gym and change what you're eating.

   There is nothing more satisfying than looking in the mirror after months of intense cardio, long high volume workouts and low macros and seeing the work looking back at you. When you can look in the mirror and see a warrior looking back at you, you will love yourself for what you are becoming.

   Don't do this for anyone else; do this because you take yourself seriously, because yourself deserves to be more powerful, sharper, leaner, bigger and stronger.

3. **"Do it because they said you wouldn't."** That's right, fuck them, you'll show them who you really are. Right now they may be saying you won't, you don't have it in you, you don't have the genetics, and you're silly. In a couple of years from now they will be asking you how you did it, and what secrets

and advice can you give them so that they, too, can do the impossible.

Tell them, "You told me I couldn't do it, that's how I did it." Let the haters and the nay sayers fuel the fire in your soul. But don't let it consume you. It doesn't matter who you are, or how much respect people have for you, or where you are right now, because you can change all that.

Every single hateful comment anyone has ever said to you should fuel you to move weights and eat to make GAINZ, and get shredded. To every single kid out there who has ever been told "you can't," prove them wrong. You can do anything you set your mind to.

Make up your mind as to when, why, and how, then execute. Shut them up and prove to yourself and anyone else that you are strong and powerful, that you do have the heart to make something of yourself.

You're more than just some kid in the world, you are a warrior. You have the mindset to do what it takes, you have the fire to tear past every goal, to eat the right foods, to train every day. One day you will look back on the day you started and get cold chills thinking how fucking awesome you have become.

4. **"Do it to be that sexy Ex GF or BF,"** seriously, whatever floats your boat. When you first go through a breakup it seems like your life is over, back to the single game again. You never thought this would be you. You thought you

were going to be married, it was a done deal, surprise muthafucka.

Your ex has a new lover and it's been less than a month, you are forgotten, old news, it's over. Does that make you mad? Well, it should. It's easy to be defeated at this point. You will be a little down on yourself and you may not think that you're good enough.

Everyone has 2 options when heart broken by the one person they gave their everything to. Option A is do nothing; go backwards in life, be sad, and lose self-worth. Option B is the clean slate, start working out, start counting macros or meal planning, or at least eating intuitively, take your goals and yourself seriously.

The great thing about new beginning's is the fact that you have a blank slate. You can start all over. You can do anything. Choose to see this as an opportunity, even in the mist of the pain and mental agony.

If you are going through something, whether it's a breakup, lost friendship, or change of career, I am glad you're reading this. I have been there. In fact, I lost them all at once, job, GF who I was ready to propose to, place of living, passion, I lost it all at once. This happened to me around the end of 2015, early 2016.

I became a bit depressed. All I had left was my passion for a health & fitness lifestyle. After a month of being broken, I picked myself up, propelled myself back into intense workouts, working out 7 days a week, and eating insane amount of food. I built a lot of muscle, made a lot of GAINZ, and it was all rooted from pain.

I was able to bring my deadlift up about 70 pounds, bench-press up around 40 pounds and squat went up around 40 pounds. Deadlift went from 365 to 435, bench-press went from 405 to 445, squat went from 405 to 445.

I had been stuck right around these strength and muscle levels for years; don't get me wrong, I always diet and workout hard, but when I lost everything all at once it awoke a fire inside me. That fire is growing stronger and stronger. The point is, whatever you're going through, you can use it as a boost of willpower.

There is no reason to be defeated when you can build yourself back up even stronger than you were before, even sharper, even more confident. Why not? If you are happy with yourself, secure with yourself, confident, determined and devoted to becoming better, this won't hurt as badly.

Become that sexy, wildly successful ex, why not? If the thought of that motivated you, act on it, get in the gym, and adopt the dieting knowledge in the book! Start setting goals in the gym, start setting goals with your strength, with your physique, with your diet, and then act on all of them and make these goals become achievements.

Just please do us both a favor and don't lose the drive and dedication as soon as you meet someone new and become a limp noodle again.

There is nothing worse than someone who thinks they can settle and be lazy because they are in a relationship. No, that's how relationships that could be good, go bad.

Once you begin eating right, and working out, it's a lifestyle, you must keep going. Going through something like a breakup is a good time to start your lifting career, as well as eating better, keeping track of what you eat, etc., but you must keep going afterwards.

After the first difficult part of the breakup starts to wear off, you must not lose that mentality of being a fighter, a warrior, changing yourself for the better, and growing. It is imperative that you continue to find powerful reasons to hit new goals in the gym, get stronger, leaner, healthier, more confident, and more powerful.

This is a never ending progression, never stop growing. If you stop growing, everything you have built will began to atrophy. You want to always be growing, be moving forward in health and fitness and in life.

5. **"I can't take being bullied anymore"** or being put down for the way I look. Whether you're being picked on for being overly skinny or overly fat, it digs at your soul, and it digs deep. As if you need to be reminded of how you look constantly, you're already killing yourself in your own head, there is no need for outside fuckery to add to the mentally agony of hating your body.

You owe it to yourself to go out there and

change your body for <u>you</u>. It sucks being picked on, but what makes it even harder are the voices in your head. If you can take control of your own mind, and use it to change, then nothing on the outside will ever effect you again.

Conquer the demons on the inside and the bullies and haters on the outside will be nothing more than ignorant people who fuel you to go harder, get stronger, and be more. Our greatest fear isn't that we couldn't do it, it's that we would somehow be in a worse situation by trying.

We think by putting ourselves out there that we will be put into more mental discomfort. I have news for you, it's all in your head. Danger is very real, fear isn't. Every worry you have that you will fail, every fear that you will look stupid, every fear of judgement by the voice in your head and by others, none of it is real.

Do you want to know what is real? Action, doing things, making things become real. Nothing is real until you make it so. You can think all you want, negative or positive, but none of it will materialize until you take action upon it. No more pain, make up your mind right now. "I will not be picked on anymore, I will become a warrior, and I will rise above all of them".

6. **"I need to do this for my family",** I must do this. It baffles me that we feel it's necessary to spend so much money on health insurance when we aren't even paying any attention to our own bodies. Change your life for your family, change your life

to lead by example. Choose to be the leader, right now.

It's imperative that we pay as much attention to our health as we do our finances. Health and fitness is a form of currency. The only true currency is time, and time is money. Your level of health and fitness directly dictates how much time you have on this earth, so health and fitness is finance indirectly.

If you develop a debilitating disease because of your lifestyle, your eating, and your sedentary ways, what will your kids have to look up to? If you're sitting on the coach all of the time watching TV, eating potato chips and ice-cream, what will your kids be learning?

If you're lazy and out of shape, who will your kids look to for health and fitness advice? It's supposed to be you! There is no need to hire any health and fitness professional if you have this book, and you have willpower. That's all you need and for a 100th of the price.

Do you want your kids to grow up with no ambition thinking it's normal to be sedentary all of the time, and eating shit? Want your kids to be picked on for being under muscled or overweight, just like you were? Want your kids to have health problems like you do? I don't think so. This is on you, if you don't take your health and fitness seriously, you're hurting your family.

If this doesn't wake you up, you will never give a shit about anything. This isn't about money, or lust, or showing off; this is about becoming stronger, more powerful, leaner, and sharper, right now.

You know what's wrong with a lot of parents these days? They've given up before they had a chance to start, there's no passion because they let life suck it from them when they were younger. It's not too late to regain your passion and nostalgia for living. This is something you must do for your family.

It's a beautiful thing to see parents active with their children, grandparents active with their grandchildren, parents and grandparents working out with their children and grandchildren. Your kids aren't going to learn about macros and micros in school, they aren't going to learn the truth about food, just bullshit about the American diet.

It's your obligation to be a leader, a warrior to blaze the trail for yours. Get up and make things happen. Take your kid to the gym with you, do it together, go grocery shopping for the food items in this book, change your diet together. I promise you, I absolutely promise you, that this will change your family's life.

7. **"Stop doing dumb shit,"** it's not going to get you anywhere. If you're between the ages of 14-21, there are a lot of influences and pressures to waste all of your time getting drunk and high. There is absolutely no reason whatsoever to get drunk at a stranger's house with a bunch of kids that have no idea what they're doing or why they're doing it.

Getting high is nothing more than a medicine; it doesn't change your life, it only covers it for a few moments. You're not cool, and you're not going anywhere. There is some bullshit stigma that all kids should be out having fun, doing dumb shit.

These are the same kids that will be under muscled and overweight at thirty with a small house and no ambition other than drinking on the weekends with their toxic bodies and going home to their overweight wives. That cycle will last the rest of their lives.

There isn't any magical lifestyle change that is supposed to happen from age 15 to 30, you are going to be the same person when you're 30 as you're becoming at this moment, just a much more prevalent version. Do yourself a favor, young one, and get a gym membership with that part-time job, and start using the diet knowledge in this book to build something out of that little body.

Let me tell you something, all of that bullshit that you think is cool in high school won't last three years. The nostalgia of getting drunk and high with your friends will die after high school along with your chance of being anything in life. If you learn to be dedicated to the gym, and to eat intuitively, and use meal plans or macros while you're young, you will have a strong foundation to build off for the rest of your life.

That great thing is that 99% of the time, someone who learns the discipline and dedication of lifting, dieting, and making GAINZ can apply that dedication and discipline to any other area of their life. The fitness lifestyle has massive carry over to every other part of your life.

You become mentally tough, consistent, sharper, quicker, and more certain in your decisions. Do you want to be a nothing in three years from now? Or do you want to be somebody? The choice is completely up to you.

Your 20's will be a product of your teens. There are tons of 21-year-olds who are built, sharp minded, great decision makers, and who are more successful than the majority of 50-year-olds. There is absolutely no reason to waste away your younger years doing pointless dumb shit when you could be building yourself and growing as a person inside and out.

For most of us, the gym and the kitchen are where our lives changed forever. One decision a day will create the rest of your life, one small step at a time. Make your parents proud, but above all, do it for you and your future. It doesn't matter where you come from, what matters is where you go.

8. **"Work out because it makes life better"**, it makes life much better. Trust me when I say this, being a stronger, leaner, sharper, and happier you is something that you want. I promise you, if you take this seriously it will drastically improve your quality and quantity of life.

We aren't designed to be sedentary, we are meant to be up and moving. We are meant to break down muscles and rebuild them stronger, we are meant to sweat, to work, grow stronger and more powerful.

Getting stronger and faster is part of fitness; progressive overload makes you better at life. Progressive overload is simple: do a little more each time you go to the gym. Lift more weight, do more reps, do more sets, take less time in between sets, slow down your reps, exaggerate the isometric (negative portion of your rep), do the lift more times per week, put more emotion into your workouts.

Those are all different ways to progress week by week, month by month. You can progress the same way with cardio on the treadmill, or the stair stepper or elliptical. You can up your MPH by .1-.2 per week, up your MPH by .25-.5 for a couple minutes of your cardio session per week, or up the intensity of the cardio session.

On the treadmill you can up the incline by 1 level each week, or more if you're feeling like putting a hurting on yourself. On the stair stepper you can add a weight jacket for a little higher resistance and on the elliptical you can up the resistance by one point per week. You can also do this in blocks, up the intensity for 5 minutes out of the 30-minute cardio session, then 10/30, 15/30, 20/30, 25/30 and then finally you have upped your entire cardio session to 30/30 over a period of 6 weeks.

There are tons of ways to progress, tons of ways to get better, tons of ways to get bigger, faster, stronger, leaner, and sharper. My suggestion to you is to get on a program. I have many; you can find programs, whether bodybuilding or powerlifting, just about anywhere.

The key is to stick to one for at least 6 months whether it's one of mine or someone else's. Here's what's awesome; you will start to notice that you are better at life. You are sharper, your mind is more clear, you have more energy all of the time, you have a higher tolerance for work, you can much more easily pick heavy things up, your work ethic is increasing, your passion for life is increasing.

BAE needs you to hold her, the whole world in your hands for a moment, you betcha, you have the strength! Need to deadlift a small car to save a small dog for that really sexy individual over there? You will be able to do so soon. When you get into a fight and you want to knock the other person out with one power punch? You will be able to do that, too.

Want to be able to go jogging with that cute girl or guy? You should be able to do that in just weeks. Want to become a writer? You will suddenly notice you're more creative, your thoughts flow better, you're more fluent, and dogs, cats and babies love you.

What is this sorcery? You know what it is, YOU LIFT, and you're making "DEM GAINZ". You will even be able to go outside and wash your own car, shirtless to get a tan. Bet you wouldn't do that before. Clean car + cardio + vitamins, it's nice.

That's not all. What will you do with your new

found confidence? Will you ask out that girl or guy that you were too shy to ask out before you became "LORD GAINZ"? Will you take that risk that could change your life, that risk you didn't have the confidence to take before?

Will you take control of your life and become a fucking boss? Damn right, you will, you will do all of those things. Working out and eating better does more than you could possibly imagine. You will understand exactly what I am saying once you, too, make health and fitness your lifestyle.

Here is one thing that may make you really happy and get you fired up, ready? Working out and eating great will skyrocket your sexual performance and pleasure. You will be able to go for hours and hours. Not only will you go for hours and hours, you will be more powerful and more fluent.

Since your body produces the same chemicals and activates the same hormones after an intense workout, and you now have intense workouts every day, hmm you see where I'm going with this, don't you? Your body will become much more efficient with these chemicals and hormones. They will be more easily elevated, and the elevation will last much longer during and after sex.

Fireworks for hours! As an effect of all this, your sex drive will go up, which also increases creativity, sharpness and alertness. Two things that are overlooked as a benefit of lifting and healthy eating are your wake and sleep patterns. Yes, you will fall asleep more easily at night, and wake up with much more energy in the morning.

It will take you much less time to get going in the morning, and much less time to go to sleep at night. It's almost like you're putting your mind and body into its natural rhythm and becoming the powerful version of yourself that you were always meant to be.

At the end of the day, working out and eating well makes every aspect of your life better, not just a couple of things, <u>everything</u>. You're in the right place to change you, to make your life amazing, you have no reason not to. If you don't completely change your life after reading this book, that's on you. Read it as many times as you need to.

9. **"Working Out Helps You to Become a Winner"** in life. If you set and achieve goals inside the gym, inside the kitchen, on the scale and in the mirror, then you can practically set and achieve goals in any area of your life. Setting and achieving goals is nothing more than a learning pattern and a character trait that can and will become a part of you.

Goal setting, and goal accomplishing is a cycle that you can and will plan for and become accustomed to. The great thing about it is, it's not hard. In fact, it's easy, and you want to do it. In my humble opinion, being honed to setting and achieving goals seems like a great thing, especially when everyone else is addicted to being lazy and floating through life.

True happiness doesn't come from eating candy, or buying things, or scratching short term itches. True happiness doesn't come from fun little nostalgic pastimes. True happiness comes from having dreams and turning those dreams into goals, and then accomplishing those goals over and over again.

True happiness comes from putting in the work, the hours, the days, weeks, months and years and seeing your work pay off. When you are getting started the victories will seem small. As you gain experience and grow, you will learn that those little wins are what create big change.

Becoming a winner is a psychological game, my friend. When you put in a lot of work and you get the results, it builds your confidence to achieve goals and win. When your brain associates "the work" with a happiness and a positive outcome, you will be eager to put in more and more work.

You will be working your ass off with a twinkle in your eye, knowing that you're becoming something; you're winning at life. The more you set and achieve goals, the more goals you make, the bigger goals you make, the more challenging goals you set for yourself, the more of an Alpha you become.

Once you start accomplishing goals, you will be addicted soon afterwards. The feeling of setting and accomplishing a goal is like no other. It's ok to fail at goals, but you need to set goals that you will be able to hit the majority of the time.

If you're hitting 75% of your goals or more, when you fail at the other 25% or less, it will just influence you to go harder, because you don't see yourself as a loser, you see yourself as a winner. The problem comes when people are always setting goals that are way out of their grip and they only achieve 25% of them. This isn't good for you.

When you're constantly losing you're confining yourself to be a loser. Set goals that can be achieved, that will be achieved, once every week or two. Set a behemoth goal and go after that goal with fire in your eyes.

When you accomplish those big goals, they're game changers; they will motivate you to take on the world. When you fail at them, it's ok because you succeeded at the other 9 goals this week. You will try again and put even more into it.

The progression of life, the grind, the growth; it's all predicated on setting and achieving goals, big and small. Nobody wakes up successful at anything - it takes hitting thousands of micro goals, hundreds of meso goals, and eventually making those large dreams a reality.

For example, if you just started lifting and you bench-press 95lbs, you want to hit 225lbs for a single. It won't happen overnight, or even in a month. For most people who aren't genetic freaks, it takes time. So you need to set micro goals, meso goals, and macro goals.

For the entire year, 225 for a single is the goal. Right now you're getting 95 for 2-3 shaky reps.

Where do you start? What should your first goal be? Your goal should be to get better at doing those 3 reps. If you can only get one set of 3 with this weight, drop the weight 10-20 pounds and get a second and third set of 3 repetitions. That first goal should be to hit at least 3 sets of 3 on bench-press, 95x3, plus 2 more sets at the same or lighter weight.

Once you hit that, go for 2 sets of 3 reps using 95x3, drop the weight and do that third set. Once you accomplish that goal, lets hit 95lbs for a 3 by 3 (3 sets of 3). Now let's work on your form. Work on keeping yourself from shaking, controlling the weight on the way down, pausing at the bottom of the rep, then power your way up. Work on your balance, keep your arms both pressing up at the same leverage.

This will be harder. Work towards getting 3 sets of 3 with 95lbs with perfect form. Once you can do that, move up in reps, work on 95lbs for sets of 4-5 reps. You will probably burn out on the first set, so drop the weight for set 2 and 3. Work towards a 5 by 5 with 95lbs.

These are micro goals, meso goals are 4-8 week goals. So you started at a shaky 95x3: in 2 months from now let's aim to get 95 for a 5 by 5 with close to perfect form. In another 2 months let's hit 95 for 8 clean reps and in another 2 months, let's work on hitting 95lbs for 10 reps.

Now that we're at about 6 months in, let's move up in weight. That would be 3 meso cycles of goals. After the 6-month mark, let's move to

135 and shoot for a set of 2 reps, or even 3 reps if possible. Use the same progression you used with 95 pounds; work on form, reps, and sets.

In another 6 months, let's aim to get 135 for 8-10 reps, 185 for 2-3, and 225 as your new max. This whole process is a macro goal. You can also call these micro, meso, and macro cycles. Micro meaning programing what happens within the week, meso meaning within 1-2 months, macro meaning the grand scheme of things, think 52 weeks for a macro cycle.

Once you get into the swing of hitting micro goals, and it becomes a way of life, you will be hitting meso goals. Then over time, you will hit your big picture goals. Once you get the hang of this whole process with lifting, dieting, and building muscle, you can utilize it in any other avenue of your life.

10. **"I Want to be Happy & Feel Good."** Ya do? Well, you're in the right place. Working out and eating better will make you feel better and happier than any depression or anxiety medication. I would know, I have taken both. I didn't actually start to feel better until I began to workout, do cardio and eat better.

Exercising increases those feel-good hormones that just make you want to give everyone hugs. It's proven that high intensity cardio modulates the brain in a very similar way to cocaine use. Once you finish an intense workout, your serotonin, dopamine and norepinephrine levels will be elevated.

All of these happy endorphins are flowing and you get to have your high without paying money, killing your brain cells, killing yourself, etc. This is a high that is just as good as, or better than, weed, close to cocaine, and it actually makes you healthier and improves brain health, and it's free.

As an athlete, what I can never understand is why people will go pay for drugs to get high, knowing that's its killing them, when you can get a workout high that inspires you and increases your life expectancy.

You may even get a bit of oxytocin elevation post workout, which is interesting. Guess what the exact hormones right after sex are? Wait for it, wait, wait. Norepinephrine, serotonin, and oxytocin, as well as those feel good endorphins and a couple of other hormones. Ironic or not?

You elevate the exact same hormones after sex as you do after a great workout. Now do you understand why we are so addicted to pre workout and crazy workouts on a daily basis? For us, it's like being high for hours not to mention the pump feels amazing. It is an addiction; the feeling, the highs, the mood enhancement.

Here is the thing, my friend: everyone is addicted to something, the question is, is your addiction helping you grow or tearing you down? My addiction is helping me grow!

Do you know what endorphins are? Endorphins basically represent self-produced morphine from a chemical standpoint. So after a workout you're getting a mixture of the same hormones that rise after sex, plus dopamine, which is what elevates after doing really good drugs.

Excuse my language kids, but a great post workout high is like you just came while finishing a very powerful drug at the same time. People that don't lift and don't do intense cardio will never understand what we're going through until they try it. We are meant to be addicted to exercise and sex, we are programmed by our chemical and hormonal breakdown to do so.

The amazing thing is you can get all of those feelings after a good workout; sex and drugs aren't always the best outlets to get your feels from. If you're single and looking to build something for yourself, working out is your best bet to get your feels. Having sex with strangers all of the time to get highs is, well, a bit dangerous. You will end up hurting people, making lots of babies and possibly getting an STD.

Obviously drugs are bad, they kill you and they take all of your money, and you will wind up in prison because of them, shall I say more? I don't need to explain why you shouldn't do drugs, just don't.

Working out and eating according to the knowledge in this book will make your life 100 times better than any exogenous substance can. Not only does working out and eating better raise these hormones to make you feel better, it also allows for better blood flow, blood pressure regulation, and ends most conditions related to blood flow problems.

Working out will also build your heart up, making your heart stronger and better able to pump blood efficiently. Working out and eating better even helps with your digestion, allowing you to feel much less bloated at any given point. All of these things give you more free energy throughout the day while greatly elevating mood, libido, helping you sleep and just helping you be a better you.

More Than 10 Reasons

At the end of the day, there are hundreds of reasons you should workout and eat well. These are just ten common and powerful reasons, but there are hundreds and hundreds of beneficial reasons to join the fitness lifestyle and start making GAINZ!

The point is, if you have at least 10 compelling, solid reasons to pull you towards working out, it will never be hard for you, even from the start. With all of those powerful reasons in mind, your workouts will have purpose, your life changes will make sense, and you will have no reason to quit.

It being too hard won't even be a thought. It's those people who walk into the gym on a whim that will never make it; they will just continue to pay their $10 a month gym membership but never show up. If your only reason for going to the gym is, "I need to lose a little weight," you know damn well you're not going to last a week.

If your reasons are, I want to live a long healthy life, be sexy, be happy, be energetic, lead by example, inspire, prove them wrong, make my family proud, make some GAINZ, make my ex jelly, get bigger, stronger, leaner, sharper - you better believe that fitness has just became BAE for life.

This whole process of building up reasons for fuel? You can use it for any avenue of life. I have been pursuing business and entrepreneurship since I was 15-16. I am 22 right now and I don't consider myself super successful yet. I work 16-20 hour days, 7 days a week. The only thing that keeps me going is the massive amount of reasons behind what I'm doing.

I can't stop; I have an obligation to you, to my family, to myself, and to the world. That's the only way to stay with something, you have to be drawn towards that something so tightly that you couldn't stop even if you wanted to.

Surround Yourself with the Change You Want to See.

If you want to get fit, get strong, become powerful, sharp and confident, you need to put yourself in an environment that fuels the evolution of such. There are many ways to do this. Consume content that helps you grow, and focus, FOCUS!

We, right now in 2016 and the years to come, are and will continue to be the biggest content consumers in the history of the word. You need to be on a content diet, just as you need to be on a food diet.

What do I mean by this? Whatever you're paying attention to, watching, and consuming on a daily basis is going to create your future. If you want to get bigger, leaner, stronger and sharper, you need to consume content that aligns with your goals.

There are 3 different ways to consume content: video, audio and reading. Obviously, you're already blazing the right trail if you're reading this, but you must look deeper into your day.

Are you by chance scrolling through Facebook and watching pointless negative shit? Are you playing random cellphone games just to pass the time? Are you watching tons of random television when you get home? Do you find yourself watching so much YouTube that you wind up on that really weird part of YouTube?

If you're doing any of these things, you probably need to go on a content diet. The first thing you need to do is stop spending too much time watching mindless shit on Facebook and stalking your ex. Neither of those things are going to help you move towards your health and fitness goals.

Secondly, minimize your Facebook use to no more than 15-20 minutes a day. Think you can pull that off? The thing is, you need to be living for you, not random Internet content. When you watch random shit all day, it's just like eating lots of empty food with no nutritional value. It's not doing anything for your mental well-being.

Facebook can be great for meeting people and for networking and communicating with family and friends, but it can also be poison. Don't get me wrong, I am not one of these extremists that says *delete your Facebook, it's terrible*. Fuck that, I love my Facebook, always will. You simply need to pay attention to how much dumb shit you're giving your attention to per day.

You need to go on a "low dumb shit" diet. Instead, follow people who inspire you, read things that vibe with you and what you want to grow into. Learn from the people that have already done it. Watch videos that inspire you enough to set your soul on fire.

If you're playing random cellphone games on your lunch break, just stop. Listen to an audio book, watch an educational YouTube video, have lunch with someone whose company you enjoy. The last thing you should ever do in life is waste away your time doing things that mean absolutely nothing, and bring you absolutely no value.

When you get home from work, I know, I know you're tired and deserve to relax. Here's the thing: I am not saying not to have fun; I am saying to pay attention to what your escapisms are.

If you're watching the Price Is Right, reality TV shows and things of this nature, you are feeding your brain low leverage content. What do I mean by low leverage? What is leverage in my context? Spending your time consuming content that is adding value to your life somehow.

Everything I watch, every person I spend time with, everything I buy, every action I take, it all vibes with the way I want my life to be in a year. If you're always consuming content that helps you grow in life, you have leverage for life, "content leverage".

I would much rather someone watch a well written TV show at night than a pointless, fake reality TV show; that sort of content breeds ignorance. Watching a really interesting TV show breeds creativity. When you do high leverage things all day, it adds up. You get sharper, more consistent, more driven, more powerful, and you continue to move forward without getting stuck.

Why is this so important to your health and fitness? Your brain is the most important part of the human body, so it deserves to be fed just as good as your changing body. Your mind must change with your body, which is the part of fitness that people don't realize. You will only take your physique so far with a low leverage mindset.

Your possibilities are endless when you surround yourself with what you want to become. Surround yourself with motivated, driven, and focused people. Your mental state will always be greatly influenced by the 5 people closest to you. If there aren't any people around who vibe with your goals and lifestyle, it's ok to be a lone wolf for now.

There aren't many people like us; we are the .01%. With that in mind, you must realize that it will be hard for you to find people compatible with you. Even if you have to be a lone wolf for a couple of years, follow your heart, follow your goals, and follow your calling. It hurts a little to be alone, it's not easy, but I absolutely promise you that it's 100% worth it.

If you never have that month or year of alone time, how will you ever be able to listen to yourself or discover yourself? Most people never know what it is they actually want, they rely on the world and society to tell them what they want and who they are.

You won't, you will be different. Does that feel good? It should feel great! The path most commonly traveled is the path to mediocracy. If you're reading this book and taking action, you will never again be mediocre, ever. Like I have said, fitness isn't just working out or eating better. It's a lifestyle and a mindset of the elite.

Fit is the mindset of someone who pushes themselves past what they may have previously thought was impossible for them. Fitness is the rising of your body, mind, heart and soul. Go make some GAINZ!

Positive Attitude

This may seem like common sense, but your way of seeing things, your way of seeing yourself and the world, is everything to your health and fitness success. The thing is, the negative person is usually spot on accurate; they always know exactly what they are capable of before they ever attempt something. Therefore, they always hit their mark.

Never more, never less. Do you know what the immediate problem of that is? They will never get ahead; they will never have any leverage to grow and get better because their accuracy is geared toward where they stand.

You can lift 225 on bench-press for 1 rep, this is something you know. You also know that bench-press is your weakness; you're going to be hitting 225 for a single for a while, and you're very accurate and spot on with that. I am not saying you're negative, but that this is a pessimistic way of thinking. You're not looking at a glass half full, you are looking at a glass frozen still - it has no room to move, no margin for error.

Sure you're accurate, sure you know yourself and your body, your weaknesses, but you know what though? FUCK YOU. You have no idea what you're capable of.

Thinking this way, you will never push yourself, never grow, never get better, because why would you even try? After all, you already know your boundaries and capabilities. You will never put 110% in because you don't believe that extra 10% is possible. You are thinking in square thoughts when success is actually an imperfect circle.

Here is the thing my friend: a loser thinks he is always right and will give up betterment to be "RIGHT". The winner knows he will be wrong 50% or more of the time and embraces that as a strength. You are powerful beyond measure and attempting to put a ceiling on your ability is wasting your potential.

There is no roof on what we are capable of, there is no ceiling on growth, and there is no wall you can't climb. Stop settling for what you think you are capable of and open up your mind and body to your full potential as a human being, or forever remain average.

Give yourself credit for the small wins, you deserve credit for those fucking wins, they're your wins! Having high standards is a good thing, but you don't have high standards if you have a highly limited perception of what you are capable of partnered with an inability to stop and appreciate the little wins, the daily growth.

The issue with thinking this way is that you will never get it, you will never be your own standard. You're never going to get there because there is no "there". The only thing that there is, is now. If you can't learn to appreciate the now, you will never realize your goals and dreams because they will always be slightly out of reach.

You will never realize how powerful you could become because you can't fathom how powerful you already are. You will never realize what you can and will do because you fail to see what you currently are doing.

It's imperative that you adopt a positive mental attitude towards yourself, your goals, your achievements and life. Most people never quite get there. Optimists are usually inaccurate; they never seem to hit the nail on the head in terms of their own capability. Their margin of error is much higher than a pessimist and they have no ego towards that fact - they don't need to be accurate.

The optimist sees him or herself better than they

actually are at all times, that's leverage for life. You always have room to grow, room to expand, room to improve and get better. The optimist will go to the gym knowing they previously hit 225 for a single, looking to hit 225 for a double. In the optimist's mind, they are about to destroy this set of 225 for 2 reps.

They may be shitty at the bench-press, but they don't see themselves as shitty, they see themselves as someone who crushes it with every opportunity they're blessed with. 225 may be very heavy for them, but they are able to bottle up every bit of pent up energy they have, and push themselves beyond what others would think they are capable of progressing to.

Basically, the optimist will look to become Super Saiyan 3. That was a Dragon Ball Z reference, if you didn't catch that. If you haven't seen DBZ, just type in *Goku transforming to SS3 for the first time* on YouTube, Goku is a fucking optimist.

The optimist is the type of crazy person who leaves nothing on the table. In fact, fuck it, they will go and get a second table, plot twist, surprise MUTHAFUCKA.

The optimist doesn't see the glass half full. We have it all wrong. They see a glass full of ice that when eating, will expend far out of the glass. But for now, it appears to be solid. Nothing is ever so black and white. There is no ceiling to the capability of an optimist; no roof, no barrier that cannot be broken.

Limitless

The optimist if fully aware of their limitless potential. Not only that, but they use that awareness to move forward at a rate 10x faster than the pessimist. They may never be spot on correct but you better believe they will keep improving because they always see themselves better than they are.

They may bench-press 225 for a single, but they will push the boundaries to 110% and they will bench-press 225 for 2 repetitions. Even if they fail the first time, they will come back in a few weeks and succeed; the success of an optimist is inevitable. There is no end point, success is a forever progression.

You must enjoy every single win and the optimist embraces this. Every win will be cherished greatly. You have high standards and you think big enough to achieve them. You will win big but understand the little daily wins are what create the macro wins!

I can always do a little more, push a little further, go a little higher, push another boundary, because I am infinitely powerful. The conception of my perception is predicated 100% on moving forward. I can never lose because I am always thinking one step ahead, I am an optimist. I always see myself just a little stronger, just a little bigger, just a little sharper, and just a little more successful than I may appear to be, and I will always grow into that vision.

The optimist and the pessimist both define themselves by the limitations and boundaries they place on themselves. The thing is, the optimist places limitations and boundaries that allow him to always have room to grow.

We must keep a positive state of mind while pursuing our health and fitness goals, or else our perception will fail to align with our goals and our destination will be unclear. You must see yourself for how powerful you are, you must see yourself succeeding, you must see yourself doing better than you already are.

Confucius said he who says he can, and he who says he can't, are both usually right. I believe that with all of my heart and soul. Your body is the canvas but your mind is the paintbrush. Your mind is the single most important part of your physique. Without the proper control of your mind, you will always be limited by your own beliefs.

If you can think any thought in the world, without restriction, why not think big, think strong, think sharp, think forward, think GAINZ. You are what you think you are, you are capable of what you allow yourself to be capable of, and you will become whatever you set out to become.

It's a simple concept at the base level, but while it is simple, we still always somehow find ourselves slipping back to habitual thinking of limitation and boundaries. The only limitation is you, get out of your own way. Limitlessness is a choice that all of us have the blessing of choosing, if we have the capacity to do so.

You are either your most powerful asset or your most destructive liability. If a goal seems big, then think big, you know what to do. Deconstruct the goal into smaller goals, lay out an action plan to hit every micro goal, every meso goal, and every macro goal this year.

If you want to lose 100 pounds you can do it. If you want to deadlift 500 pounds, plan it out. If you want to build 10 pounds of lean muscle mass, do it. It is all yours for the taking, the only thing left for you is to see it, believe it, and then achieve it.

My friend, never say it's too good to be true, never ever say that because it is true. Take this moment to think, take it all in, this is your life, take control if it, this is your mind. Guide it in the right direction. These are your goals and dreams so FUCKING MAKE THEM HAPPEN!!!

You have nothing to lose but everything to gain. Don't let one more second pass you by thinking you can't, or limiting yourself. This is your moment, all it takes is one moment to change your entire life for good, this is yours.

They say it takes some people 10 years to make a change, to take a chance. I call bullshit. It took those people 10 years to get to their breaking point; it took them 1 second to change their lives forever. You don't need 10 years my friend, all you need is this one second. Forget about everything else, FUCK IT, this is your FUCKING moment. Go make some FUCKING GAINZ!!!

CONCLUSION

I never aimed to show you the perfect diet. My goal was not to sell you on a product. I did not try to get you on my bandwagon.

The purpose of this book is to open your eyes. Making GAINZ, dieting, working out, the fitness lifestyle, so it's not so black and white. It's completely different for everybody. We all have different bodies, different minds, and different goals. We all react completely differently to foods macronutrients and micronutrients.

We all have our own perception of what to take from this book. I am not here to give you my biased opinion on anything, but just to put the facts in your face and tell you what you need to hear, not what you want to hear, not what makes me money, not what is marketable.

You are here because you wanted and deserved to make a change, and now my friend, you will. There is so much to macronutrients, fat, carb, protein, and alcohol. We need to know and understand all of them on a molecular level to be able to understand how they work for us.

Some of us do better on meal plans, others with IIFYM, and some people get their best results following Intuitive Eating. I am not here to tell you which one you should do, but to sway you in the right direction according to you, your lifestyle, your goals, your mind and your body.

For any program or person to tell you that one way of eating is the best way, is just wrong, they are trying to market to you their product. But you know the truth. The method and structure that is best for me is the structure and method that fits me, personally.

There is a lot of bullshit out there, like fitness myths, skewed perceptions, ignorant states of mind, etc. Luckily, you now have the power to stop all of those bullets from touching you, for you now know what's real, you know what's true. You're in control of your own mind, your own body, and your own health and fitness destiny.

You have unlimited potential to become something others will only dream of becoming. So go out there and make your dreams come true, just DO IT, JUST FUCKING DO IT, MAKE YOUR DREAMS COME TRUE.

The end.

MYFITNESSPAL HACKS

MyFitnessPal is the most well-known fitness app for macronutrient tracking. This is the app that I have used personally to consistently hit my target macronutrient numbers daily. This app has been a crucial tool leading me into natural bodybuilding contests.

MyFitnessPal did it right, so right, that UnderArmour bought them out a couple of years ago. Using MyFitnessPal, you are able to document each day tracking your fat, carbs, protein and overall caloric intake.

MyFitnessPal has changed a lot over the years; as an online fitness coach, this app is my main tool to teach clients how to count their macro nutrient intake. I decided to write this book for my clients as well as anybody else out there looking to count macros, or just become more efficient and effective with MyFitnessPal.

1-GETTING SET UP

Entering Starting Stats

There are a couple of ways to get started; enter everything manually, use email, or use Facebook. As with any other app, using your Facebook to quick add all of your data makes things move a lot quicker and smoother in the sign-up process. Just always make sure that you are not allowing the app to post on your behalf on Facebook. The only things you will need to enter from there is your activity level, current bodyweight, and weight loss goals. Ok, your profile is setup, now it's time to configure it.

Sharing & Privacy, Diary Settings

Go to the more tab, then settings.
Sharing & Privacy- *Go to the more tab, then settings, sharing & privacy.*

- *News Feed Sharing-* Make sure to take a second to check everything you would like to share. If there is anything you want to keep to yourself, uncheck it. These boxes will all be checked as part of the default settings, so everyone will see everything. If you're not ok with that, then go and uncheck the boxes you aren't comfortable with.

- *Diary Sharing-* Choose to share your diary with all of the public, only your friends, to have a private diary, or to lock your diary with a key password that you yourself give people. P.S., if you become YouTube famous, you could charge people for your MyFitnessPal diary key. Do not misunderstand me - I am not saying you should, just that you could if your diet was that cool. But your diet is probably not that fucking cool.

- *Email Settings-* Choose to receive the MyFitnessPal Newsletter and if you would like people to be able to find you by your email address. There is an entire assortment of slider options under the first 2, slide them to your liking. All of these sliders relate to the social aspect of MyFitnessPal, so use them to your advantage; if you are using the app solely for counting macros, I would turn most of them off.

- *Apple Health Kit for IOS-* I personally have an iPhone, so if you do happen to have an android, there may be a very similar app. The Apple Health Kit is an app that allows you to connect and integrate your fitness apps together, making it easier to track your fitness lifestyle. If you decide to download the Apple Health Kit app, after you open it, tap the source icon and select MyFitnessPal to give the app permission to sync up.

- *Facebook Sharing-* Allow your Facebook friends to find you, and choose if you want MyFitnessPal to post auto updates on your Facebook. Personally, I would tell you not to allow the app to post any auto updates because it will probably spam your Facebook with your diary data and weigh ins.

- Ad Settings & Passcode- you will have ads either way, so don't even worry about this, and you don't need a settings passcode, no need for that nonsense. I don't even know why that setting is there.

***Diary Settings*-** *Go to the more tab, then settings, then diary settings.*

There are a few different settings in the diary settings tab, so here is the quick description of the settings and what they do.

1. *Show All Meals in Diary Tabs*- this slider is pretty straight forward, either choose to show the individual meals in your diary tab or not.

2. *Use Multi-add By Default*- this slide allows you to be able to add multiple food items at once.

3. *Show Diary Food Insights*- this slider, when turned on, gives you little insights like how much saturated fat is in a food or the amount of sugar.

4. *Default Search Tabs*- choose your default search tab. You have the option to choose between recent, frequent, my foods, meals or recipes. This is something I would personally leave as recent while learning the app. Once you get in the rhythm of eating frequent foods, then change the default search tab (DST) to frequent. Down the road, you can change it to any of the other DST's, but I have found these two to be the most useful.

Weekly Nutrition Settings *Go to the more tab, then settings, weekly nutrition settings.*

This tab allows you set your week to start on a specific day but it will be preset to 7 days ago. This is the amount of data that will be displayed on your nutrition report. If you want to look at data from one day or collectively from 7 days, you can do that with this setting.

Push Notifications *Go to the more tab, then settings, Push Notifications.*

Check all the boxes that you would like to allow the

app to notify you of. Personally, I would leave most of them unchecked except the goal oriented notifications.

Steps *Go to the more tab, then steps.*

You have the option here to either use your cellphone's or tablet's built in motion processor which will be preset, or to choose an app to set up your footstep tracking. You also have a setting for daily step goals which can be set to any goal number you want.

2-DIARY HACKS

Diary

The diary is arguably what makes MyFitnessPal so good. You start out with 4 meals:

1. Breakfast
2. Lunch
3. Dinner
4. Snacks

Basically, everything about these 4 meals is customizable. Here you a have a powerful platform to create your own diet.

Meal Names & Amounts

For this option, go to the website version because it's easier to change meal names and the amount of meals on the website version.

Go to food, then settings, and there you can change the name of your meals or the amount. Here are my meals.

1. Maybe
2. Yas Lunch Time

3. Nope I'm at the Gym

4. Time for a Samach

5. Before Bed Sweet Snack

6. Fatass

+ Add Food

This is where things get interesting and it's also where you need to pay attention.

Search for a food- Here you can type in any food item and MyFitnessPal will display the results. You can type anything in and you will get tons of results, just like a Google search, but for food with macros.

You can place this food item in any of your meals. The meal will list its fat, carbs, protein, fiber, and all of the micronutrients. Once you add the item into your diary, it will display how many calories, macros and micros you have left for the day to hit your target. You can add as many food items to one meal as you like, within reason.

Search for a Food- Restaurants

MyFitnessPal has just about every single franchised restaurant in their database. If you want to track any meal at a franchised restaurant, just type in the name of the restaurant and then the meal you ordered. It's that simple. Now add it to the applicable meal. Here are some examples.

1. Cookout Cheeseburger- 578 calories, 40.8 fat, 21.7 carbs, 29.2 protein.

2. Olive Garden- Salmon Bruschetta- 1,110 calories, 54 fat, 78 carb, 70 protein.

3. Chipotle Chicken Burrito- 580 calories, 17 fat, 79 carbs, 27 protein.

If your goal is to lose weight, remember chefs don't weigh their food, so don't expect to be super accurate. I recommend that you learn the average size of the meals you get on a consistent basis. To be safe, always round up a little bit on the meal size, 1.25 to 1.5 if the meal seems huge. The serving size will be preset to 1.0, so you have to be honest with yourself here.

If at a restaurant like Chipotle where there are several options, I recommend you watch them add each topping to your food and add them in separately because just entering in burrito or bowl is going to be extremely inaccurate.

Olive Garden, or any fancy Italian restaurant for that matter, usually gives you a shit ton of food, so I would estimate way up at a place like this.

Fast food places like Cookout are pretty standard on their serving sizes, so you're a little safer there in terms of accuracy, but not in terms of fat content or overall calories.

The point is, you can eat wherever you want, but play smart, in accordance to your goals.

Unfranchised restaurants are a little more difficult but manageable. Here's what you do at an unfranchised restaurant: type in the food items you ordered, find the highest calorie version of the food item, and add it to the applicable meal. Be sure to check the macros on whatever you add; if the macros are way off, through the stratosphere, a troll probably created it. Find something that seems accurate and add that - after doing this for a while it becomes intuitive.

Barcode Scanning

You can scan any food with a barcode and it will enter into your diary. Make sure that when doing this, you check the amount of serving sizes in the food item and make sure you have the correct amount entered for the meal you are about to eat. If you decide to eat less than the entire food item, it's your job to weigh it out on a food scale - you can be highly accurate that way.

Weighing in grams

Here is a list of food items that should be weighed in grams:

1. Fruits
2. Vegetables
3. Leaves
4. Rice
5. Pastas
6. Beans
7. Oats

Anytime you weigh in grams, you will be much more accurate than ounces, but it's not 100% necessary for everyone.

The first thing you need to do is go on Amazon and purchase a food scale. Here is a link.

You can get a nice food scale for $10, so I don't want to hear any financial excuses.

Let's first go into how to weigh your fruit and veggies.

With whole fruit and veggies, turn your scale on, set the units to grams, ensure the scale is set to 0 grams, and place your food item on the scale.

Open MyFitnessPal, go to your diary, and find the meal you would like to enter the food item in. Whatever it is you're eating, some sort of apple or vegetable, type it in in the search bar. Once you have the food, pop up pick one and change the serving size to grams; enter the applicable amount of grams in number of servings.

Another way you can do it is to type in (food item) 100g.

Example- Fuji Apple 100g

Here are a few examples of how you would enter this in the serving size:

So you just weighed your Fuji Apple and its weight is 101 grams. Your serving size should be 1.02 based off a 100g serving size.

Here are 3 more examples just so you're clear.

1. Banana 127g = serving size of 1.27

2. Blueberries 154g = serving size of 1.54

3. Big Cucumber 205g = serving size of 2.05

Again these examples are all based on you typing in 100g after your food item.

Create a New Food

When you click 'add food' in your diary, you have a few different tab options; you have Recent, Frequent, My foods, Meals and Recipes. One inch under those options you have the "create a new food" box, click that box.

On the first page, you have the option to enter a brand name, description, serving size, or servings per container.

Please be precise and honest here - the data you're entering could either help lots of people or hurt lots of people. On the second page you have a page of data to fill out; fill out as much data as possible so that you can be accurate when logging this food in the future; also so that others can use it to their advantage - this is a give and take community.

Restaurant Logging

This is by far the most powerful update MyFitnessPal has done since its launch.

When MyFitnessPal created this option, they had a goal in mind! The goal MyFitnessPal was looking to achieve was to help users become more effective at counting macros while eating out.

LEARN / MYFITNESSPAL UPDATES / PRODUCT NEWS / MARCH 21, 2016

MyFitnessPal Restaurant Logging: Now on iOS and Android

MyFitnessPal stated in the above blog post that a restaurant menu item is logged every 3.2 seconds in their app. Interestingly, they found that one of the biggest pain points of their users has been making good decisions while eating at restaurants.

Here is what they found in a recent survey.

- Nearly half of all MyFitnessPal's users eat out at least once per week.

- Well over 80% of these users find it tough to make healthy food decisions while eating out.

- Almost 80% would always look at the nutrition info before they ordered, if that info were available.

This is when the *Restaurant Logging Feature* was born!

Here are 3 main features that MyFitnessPal outlines on their above blog post:

- Efficiently log restaurant items without having to search the database.

- View the calorie and nutrition data from the menus of 500,000 restaurants nationwide.

- Call up the diet gods of MyFitnessPal to pull you up a map of the nearby restaurant menus at first glance so you can see which options best fit your macros for the day. Wow, that is helpful.

To get to restaurant logging, go to diary, + add food to the applicable meal, then click the map symbol in the top right corner (IOS). Now that you are there, click the magnifying glass in the top right corner; type in your current location and press search. Now you should have an assortment of restaurants to choose from.

If the restaurants have a green check beside them, you can click them and view their entire menu; at any point while viewing a particular website's menu, you can go ahead and add a food item to your meal. The restaurant choices without menus have not put out their nutrition info yet. The cool thing is when you click them you can then directly request for that restaurant to send MyFitnessPal their menu and nutrition data by clicking 'request'. Once you have clicked request, you have 3 options.

1. Push Notification

2. Email

3. Don't notify me

Which option you choose is entirely up to you. Personally I would like to be notified once the restaurant has published their menu.

I have been in the macro game for 3+ years now and I can tell you one thing - the more food options, the easier it is to stay consistent and adhere to your macros.

Create a New Recipe

To get to create a new recipe go to diary, + add food to the applicable meal, recipes, then click create a new recipe.

Now you have 2 options - add from the web or enter ingredients manually.

If you choose add from the web, MyFitnessPal gives you a list of recipe websites to pick from; pick a website, go find something you like, and import the ingredients. When you choose to import something you found on one of the featured websites, it simply lists all ingredients in an organized fashion and allows you to copy and paste them onto your database.

The other option is to enter the ingredients manually. You would use this option if you were looking to create a dish, or a meal, dip, sauce, etc. You could also use this option to manually enter any cookbook recipes.

When manually adding a recipe, you have the title, servings, and bulk import option.

- Title is the name of the recipe you either found or created.

- Servings are the amount of total servings in the recipe item.

- If you choose to bulk import ingredients, enter one ingredient per line, add as many as you want, and MyFitnessPal will search its database and match all of your ingredients and automatically make a list of every item; this list is ready to go with calories and macros.

You can also choose to search them independently after clicking on to the next page.

This brings you to the save recipe page - only thing left to do here is to check and see if everything looks right. Make sure the servings are right, title is spelled correctly, and the macro numbers look on point. From here you can choose to either save your recipe, or save it and log it.

Quick Add

To get to quick add, go to diary, + add food to the applicable meal, quick add.

This option allows you to quickly add calories to a meal. You do need the premium version to be able to actually add the macronutrients. Since the premium version is currently $10 a month, it would only make sense for you to purchase the premium version if you would personally receive high value from most of the premium options. Otherwise, I would just stick to all of the other options that don't require the premium version.

3-MyFitnessPal Hacks

Diary- Exercises

If you go down to the bottom of your diary you will find the exercise tab. You have a couple of different options here, so let me break them down.

Step Calorie Adjustment (iPhone) If you have an Android, you will have a similar measurement app appear here.

Once you click step calorie adjustment you have a couple of different options; you can either click calorie adjustment or learn more.

- *Calorie Adjustment-* MyFitnessPal pulls your personal calorie burn directly from their total diary calorie App Gallery partners. One thing you want to make sure of if you do set up calorie adjustment, is syncing the time zone of MyFitnessPal with your partner device. This little partnership allows the step counting app to communicate with MyFitnessPal and adjust your daily calorie goals accordingly.

   My recommendation? Using this tool will overcomplicate your life. I am not telling you not to use it, just that personally, it's too much for me. However, this is definitely a cool little option if you're into recording every little bit of data you can. This could help you, but if you're a normal busy individual, this could overwhelm you.

- *Learn More FAQ-* If you want to really learn everything about calorie adjustment, just go to the FAQ page and dive in.

- *App Gallery-* MyFitnessPal has this miraculous little gallery of apps that highlights the many apps and products that can be linked to your account to enhance and expand your user experience with MyFitnessPal.

   There are tons of cool apps that will be sure to tickle your fancy, so go check them out and create your own personal MyFitnessPal experience. If you want to check out these apps, go to the "more" tab on your cellular device and then click "Apps & Devices." If you want to view these apps on the MyFitnessPal website, simply click the apps tab and boom, I give you the "App Gallery."

+ Add Exercises

You will find this option at the bottom of your exercise tab on the diary page. Now you have 2 options, cardio and strength.

- *Cardio-* When you click cardio, you will now have 3 tabs: history, my exercises and all exercises. Once you have some exercises in your diary, your history will start to fill up with cardio.

- *My Exercises* gives you the options to quickly create and add your own custom exercises. Click create a new exercise and go for it. Once you're on the new exercise page, enter your description, calories burned and start time; boom - you have entered a cardio exercise into your cardio diary.

- *All Exercises-* This gives you a list of just about every cardio exercise you can imagine; it's basically a menu of cardio exercises you can log into your daily cardio diary.

- *Strength –* You have the same tabs as you do with the cardio page but my exercises and all exercises will be different.

- *My Exercises* gives you the option to add a description of your exercise along with the number of sets, reps and weight. This is a great tool for anyone recording their workout who's using any sort of progression scheme. You could use this as a tool to document your workout, along with the individual exercises, reps, sets, and weight. Recording your numbers is very important because it gives you something to go on week after week.

- *All Exercises-* This gives you a list of just about

every strength exercise you may be doing - it's basically a menu of strength training exercises you can log into your daily strength diary. If the strength exercise you are performing isn't there, add it!

- *Tracking Strength exercises using My Exercises-* I would consider this to be one of the greatest exercise hacks of MyFitnessPal. If you are a coaching client of mine or just about any other online coach, you will be recording every lift; you will be recording the weight, sets and reps. It looks like this: Weight x Sets x Reps. For example: Bench-press: 275x5x5 which breaks down to 275 for 5 sets of 5 reps. Now let me show you how you can enter that into your Exercise Diary.

+ Add Exercise- More

To the right, inside the + add exercise tab you will find the "more" side tab. Clicking the more side tab will pull up 3 options.

1. *Manage Step Tracking-* This option takes you to a page where you can set up your mobile phone to use its preset step tracking motion processor, connect a new device or app with MyFitnessPal for step tracking, or choose not to track steps. You can also enter your daily step goals on this page.

2. *View Partner Apps-* On this page you can view all of MyFitnessPal's partnering apps and devices.

3. *Copy from Date-* This option allows you to carry over exercise data from a previous date and automatically paste it into today's exercise diary.

Nutrition & Notes

You will find these 2 rectangle shaped tabs at the bottom of your diary page. Let me tell you what they do.

Nutrition gives you 3 different slider pages to view your nutrition data from. You have calories, nutrients and of course macros. The calories slide gives you a pie chart containing the amounts of all your meals out of 100%.

You can toggle between a day view, week view, or pick a date, any date since you started, and view the meal data from that date. The nutrition slide gives you a macro and micronutrient breakdown of where you are for the day and also how many macros and micros you have left.

Just like the first slide, you have the choice of viewing today's data, this week's data or any day of your choice. The third slide, "macros," displays your macronutrient ratios on a pie chart just as the meal chart did for your meals. You have the same 3 toggle views as the first 2 slides.

Premium

Is premium right for you? $10 a month is a lot, in my opinion. I love MyFitnessPal, but I would have to think very carefully about that extra $10 a month, personally.

The three things that MyFitnessPal states that are the major benefits of premium are the ad-free version, better tools and better analytics.

There are many more benefits, some of which I think are very helpful. Let's dive into premium!

Macronutrients by Gram- For anyone that's serious about counting macros and building a macro plan tailored to them, it's easy to understand how important being able to pick your own macros by the gram is. Ratios aren't bad by any means but choosing your own macro numbers is far superior to choosing ratios of macros. This option alone was helpful when first released, although by itself is not worth $10 a month.

Add Daily Goals- This option allows you to add different macronutrient goals by day. You can add specific calorie and macronutrient goals for each and every day. I like goals, and I believe this can be an extremely useful tool for anyone with a set deadline for their weight loss. Goals are crucial; having goals allows you to accomplish small achievements every day reaffirming to yourself that you're doing the damn thing. This is definitely a helpful tool!

Restaurant Macro Filter- When you use the restaurant logging tool, this allows you to filter your nearby restaurant results based on your macros. In my opinion, this tool is probably the most valuable premium tool of them all. You can filter restaurants based on the levels of fat, carbs, and protein in their meals.

For you, this means you'll understand and become much more efficient at eating out at restaurants that agree with your macros. When you're looking at the menu in a restaurant, you can get very accurate with filtering the macros for your macro goals for that given day.

Quick Add Macros- This gives you the ability to quick add your macros as opposed to quick adding just calories. If you're someone who sometimes forgets what they ate and then you add them on a whim as you're falling asleep at night, this feature may help you.

Your Food Ranking- This feature allows you to see

which of the foods you eat that rank highest in calories. Understanding what foods you're eating that are highest in calories every day and historically, can help you better understand your eating habits and improve them over time. Your food can also be ranked by nutrient level, which is educating you on which foods provide the best bang for your buck regarding nutrients.

Eating more nutrient dense foods over time will help keep you fuller, keep you happier and take your health to another level. You can even rank your food based off of macros. This means ranking foods high in fat, protein, and carbs. If you're someone that is learning their body, catching their habits and completely transforming their life, this premium option may be starting to make sense for you!

Nutrition Dashboard- This allows you to change your home screen goal box at the top of your home screen. The default settings are set to show your calorie goals for the day. This feature gives you some different options to personalize your unique goals.

- *Macronutrients-* Yes, you can display your macros on the home screen box, also current macros, goals and how many you have left.

- *Heart Healthy-* You also have the option to show how heart healthy your day is going. This option displays your fat, sodium, cholesterol and calories remaining.

- *Low Carb-* This view displays your carbs, sugar, dietary fiber and calories remaining for the day.

- *Custom Summary-* Select any 3 nutrients to track and boom - you have a custom home box. You can choose to track whatever 3 things you want to track; this is entirely up to you.

Exercise Calories Settings- Decide whether or not to increase daily calorie goals when you exercise. Basically, when you burn calories doing a workout or physical activity, you can choose to let it change your daily calorie goals; meaning eat more macros or keep them the same. Personally, I don't want my macros to change every day depending on my physical activity level that day.

Is Premium for Me?

If you're someone that is new to the game and looking to learn as much about yourself, your habits and food, then premium may be worth the $10. If you travel a lot for your job or business, then 100% premium would be of high value to you for the fact that you're always eating in different locations.

If you are looking for a nutritionist but don't have the money to spend on something of that caliber, then the premium version for $10 a month would be a great bang for your buck. I also coach diet, nutrition and training if that's something you would like to learn more about click here.

The premium version is not for the dabbler, don't waste your money. Don't get the premium version before you understand how to take full advantage of everything the free version has to offer; if you're not consistently using the app, don't purchase premium.

I am someone that strategically thinks about every expense as to how much value it can provide me. If a product that costs $10 a month can provide me with $100+

a month of value in terms of time saved and knowledge learned, then buying that product is a no-brainer.

On the other hand, if you're going to dabble on the app and only receive cents on the dollar in terms of value, stay away from premium until you're ready to get a little more out of it. At the end of the day, this is a great app and it serves a different purpose for everybody; what you use it for is completely up to you. Premium is your decision - invest wisely.

4-SEVEN THINGS I LOVE ABOUT MYFITNESSPAL

1. **Diary** - The diary is what made MyFitnessPal so great and what will always make it great! You have your meals and your exercises - this is where the majority of your time on MyFitnessPal will be spent. Logging your macros. MyFitnessPal still does this better than any other fitness app in my opinion; my meals are Maybe, Yas Lunch Time, Nope I'm at the gym, Time for a samach, before night sweet snacks, and Fatass.

2. **Restaurant Logging** - The fact that you can find restaurants based off of your macros (and every restaurant has a menu with macros found by clicking that restaurant) is amazing. Counting my macros while eating out during my last contest prep was the one irritating part of the prep. Restaurant logging solves that little irritation. Restaurant logging is cool; restaurant logging is a game changer.

3. **My Exercises** - Being that I am a natural bodybuilder, I track my exercises by weight, sets,

and reps on a daily basis. I use a paperback diary to log them, and I have used google spreadsheets in the past to log both my workouts and my client's workouts. MyFitnessPal, since it's a mobile app, the same mobile app we count our macros on, is arguably faster and more convenient than both a paperback diary and a Google spreadsheet. I am not saying MyFitnessPal is the greatest resource to log your macros, but that it is now a reputable resource that has its own advantages.

4. **Create a New Food** - At any point, if you see a food that isn't in MyFitnessPal's database, you can create it right on the spot; food name, description, macros, calories and nutrients can be entered in less than 5 minutes, creating your own food. This is one of the biggest ways that MyFitnessPal has grown and thrived, by allowing users to take the wheel and create content.

5. **Community** - The evolution of MyFitnessPal has led to a highly community-driven user experience. MyFitnessPal started out with 1 goal in mind: to create the greatest fitness app on the market regarding usability and community.

When MyFitnessPal had its humble beginning, it was known for counting macros and creating foods, plus its extensive MyFitnessPal database that made flexible dieting much easier. Now it feels like more of a platform with community challenges, food and recipe creation by the user, exercise creation, blogging, and MyFitnessPal even has its own community page.

6. **Barcode Scanning** - Barcode scanning food

labels and having them ready to enter into your diet is a life saver. Any time I am scanning a food item into my diary, I can rest assured knowing that it will most likely be in MyFitnessPal's database and will pull up on my cell phone in seconds.

7. **Steps** - Once step tracking became mainstream and popular on cellular devices as well as on smart fitness gear, MyFitnessPal did not hesitate to integrate step tracking into their app. You can either use your phone's built-in step processor, connect another step tracking app to MyFitnessPal, or connect to your fit gear of choice.

5-FIVE THINGS I HATE ABOUT MYFITNESSPAL

1. **Premium** - I love the idea of premium, and I must say premium was much overdue and is well worth it for some people. However, for the majority of individuals that don't use every single feature the app has to offer, $10 a month is a bit pricey. It's hardly justifiable for the majority of people that don't count their macros 24/7, year-round.

   $3 a month would be a great price in my opinion; that would be a more valuable price for the majority of users. Either way, this is a bold and brave move by UnderArmour.

2. **Apps & Devices** - As if MyFitnessPal wasn't becoming sophisticated enough, now we have a plethora of apps to choose from. Trying to use and understand every setting and option on this app is already a handful; having a ton of other apps and

devices linked to MyFitnessPal makes it feel like it's trying to be the "Facebook of fitness apps," when I think it would be better as "the Snapchat of fitness apps."

3. **Needs Better Food Creation Vetting** - It would be shockingly easy to sabotage new MyFitnessPal users by spamming incorrect macros all over their search engine if you wanted to. You can pretty much enter anything into their database with any sort of macros, and it's not really vetted well.

    If I'm a new MyFitnessPal user, I may actually believe that giant bowl of lasagna and meatballs only had 800 calories, 100 grams of protein, 50 grams of carbs, and 22 grams of fat. When in reality the protein is probably half that with the fat doubled and the carbs tripled. Things that don't add up should be vetted and deleted more consistently.

4. **Shop Fitness Gear** - I love MyFitnessPal, but with a premium version plus a link to UnderArmour clothing, it's starting to feel much less personal and much more like a premium marketplace for fewer people. If you're just using the app to count macros, then you probably aren't also looking to buy clothing, just to count macros and learn your body.

5. **Becoming too Complex** - It's easy to reminisce about the old days when MyFitnessPal owned MyFitnessPal; I was able to count macros with nothing more than the occasional ads. I understand that banner ads and pre-role ads aren't as efficient

as they used to be regarding ad revenue, but MyFitnessPal is getting really cluttered.

I miss the purity and simplicity of the original version that MyFitnessPal represented. Now we have premium, app affiliates, steps per day, UnderArmour sales plugins, affiliate devices, challenges, blogging, etc. The point is, if anything more is added to this app I believe it would be running too far from its roots.

Conclusion - MyFitnessPal Hacked

There are so many people, both my clients and many others, who are either counting macros or looking to count macros. This book was put together for both new users of MyFitnessPal and people that already use it who would like to become a little more efficient with the app.

MyFitnessPal is a great app for anyone looking to get into the fitness community and learn their body, learn about food, and have a place to set and achieve goals. The thing is, MyFitnessPal has become a huge platform and there is a lot to learn about the app; this book is the fast track for not only learning how to use MyFitnessPal, but ultimately understanding how you can leverage the app to produce optimal results in your life.

After reading this book, you should know what practical use MyFitnessPal has for you and how to become a MyFitnessPal practitioner. This app can be a very powerful tool if understood and used to your personal advantage. Now it's up to you to put MyFitnessPal to work in your life.

21 MYTHS OF THE FITNESS INDUSTRY

Myth #1

"Fasted cardio burns more fat."

It doesn't matter what time you do cardio. Morning, midday, evening, night - burning calories is burning calories. Don't stress out about what time you do your cardio, just do it. At the end of the day burning 400 calories on the treadmill is burning 400 calories on the treadmill. Your body doesn't care what time you burn these calories.

Theoretically, it does make sense: when there's no food in your stomach, then you can burn fat stores instead of carbs. Well, there are two problems with this theory; first of all, if that were the case, you would also burn some muscle, not good. The other problem is that weight loss is about your total macro energy expenditure vs. total energy consumed in calories.

At the end of the day, you are expending more calories than if you had been sedentary by doing cardio. The timing of your cardio is completely irrelevant when it comes to basic fat loss. Fit your cardio in when it works for you. Don't stress the timing, just get it done.

Myth #2

"Not eating breakfast is bad."

No, it's not. Eating breakfast isn't going to change the amount or speed of weight you lose. Eating breakfast does not jumpstart your metabolism. I am not telling you not to eat breakfast; I am telling you that it's not a big deal.

Consider this, if you're eating 2000 calories in one day, it's always going to be 2000 calories. If you consume 2000 calories including breakfast, or you skipped breakfast and still ate 2000 calories, you still ate 2000 calories on that day. There is no science to back this myth up, only bogus studies that don't prove anything.

If you like to eat breakfast, eat breakfast; if you don't like to eat breakfast, don't eat breakfast. Bear in mind I'm not telling you a calorie is a calorie; you still need to take into account proper macronutrient ratios and eat a diet based off of 80-95% unprocessed nutrient dense food.

Myth #3

"Eating more meals throughout the day will turn on your metabolic furnace."

No, no, no. Eating every 3 hours doesn't speed up your metabolism, it just makes you anti-social. The amount of meals you eat isn't going to change the rate at which your metabolism expends calories.

Let's look at this from a base level; we have protein, carbs, and fat as fuel sources. The way we lose weight is by manipulating these 3 macronutrients; i.e. dropping caloric intake. It's not about when you eat, it's about what you eat and how much you eat.

Creating consistent meal times and planning them around your day will help you spend more time on living life and less time trying to decide when to eat or put meals together; this is more for balance in life than metabolism or fat loss.

Eat the amount of meals that makes you happy at the times that best suit your schedule, end of story.

Myth #4

"You need to eat certain "clean foods" to lose weight."

While it is healthier to eat "clean food," it doesn't do anything noticeable to your weight loss. You can eat really healthy and also be really fat; you can eat shitty and be very lean and fit. The key is to be fit and healthy, not just fit or healthy.

Regarding fat loss, a carb is a carb, fat is fat, and protein is protein. If you hit your target numbers regarding your program, and you're on a caloric deficit, you will lose weight. You should still eat 80-95% clean foods for your own health and longevity, but not specifically to lose weight.

Think of it this way, macronutrients dictate how you perform, change and lose or gain weight day to day. Micronutrients keep you healthy over the long run. It's important to make healthy food choices but the difference between health and weight loss are often misunderstood.

The point I am trying make is that you should eat mostly healthy foods, but you still need to pay attention to the amount and be consistent on the amounts. There is no reason to be a clean food robot. If you want something less nutrient dense and more for enjoyment every once in a while, eat it and don't feel bad about it. You're not doing anything wrong, you're not cheating; you're being human.

Myth #5

"You can change your metabolism in weeks."

You're out of luck. Your metabolism is your metabolism. Everyone has something called a BMR (Basal Metabolic Rate) and you can't change it in a matter of weeks. Your BMR is how many calories you burn while at rest. What you're actually doing by working out, doing cardio, and taking fat burners, is expending more calories. You're not "increasing your body's ability to burn fat."

Now, you can raise your metabolism over time by building muscle and lifting more weight in the gym; however, that doesn't happen in weeks. What people actually mean to say is that you can burn more calories doing more physical activity in the short term.

Building your metabolism is a long term journey of muscle and strength building. One could argue that it actually means to change your metabolism and technically, when you start weight training, you are making hormonal changes. These hormonal changes can be looked at as a metabolic adaptation. But I don't like to call them that simply because you could lose that increased calorie burning effect in a week if you stopped weight training prematurely.

Once you have been weight training for months and months, you will be able to increase your metabolic rate! Yes, you can alter your metabolism, but it's a long-term game, my friend. Eventually you can completely change your body chemistry so you do have some awesome stuff to look forward to!

Myth #6

"Weight loss is linear."

First of all, get that word linear out of your head. Nothing you're working towards in life will ever be accomplished in a linear progression. Success isn't linear, weight loss isn't linear. You may lose 1 pound overnight and then not lose another pound for 7 days. Or you may lose 2 pounds and then gain back .5 pounds to a pound tomorrow.

You just can't look at weight loss from a day to day window. When analyzing your weight loss progress, you need to base your success off your overall trend which should be trending down over time.

Think about this: you eat slightly different meals every day, i.e. your food weight and volume fluctuates; you eat at different times every day, drink different amounts of water each day, have more or less food in your digestive system each day, hold more or less water in your system depending on the timing of your water consumption in coordination to your weigh in.

Be patient and don't make brash diet changes when your weight is stagnant or fluctuates up and always remember, weight loss is undulating, not linear.

Myth #7

"The cave man, low carb, organic, super metabolic enhancement diet that all the movie stars used."

This is going to be a bit of a handful, so please stay with me here.

There are no one size fits all special diets that everyone uses to lose weight quick or lose weight in specific areas of the body. Special food selective or macronutrient selective/discriminative diets are all highly marketed shiny objects based on highly manipulated results and information.

It's never good to say fat, carbs, or protein are bad because you should consume all of them. Your body will adapt to just about any diet you put it on, so in theory, and on some level, any fad diet will yield some results.

Please don't get it twisted - these are short term results that will fade as soon as you end your fad diet. These diets also attempt to limit food choices or point out certain foods as bad, which is simply not the case. You can't just simply call a food bad without looking at the context of the statement. Fad diets are nothing more than sexy, manipulated info with big marketing.

Myth #8

"Carbs make you fat."

This is one of the oldest myths in health and fitness but some people still believe that the only way to lose weight is by cutting their carbs, sadly.

Yes, when you drop carbs and up protein a little you will lose weight, but that isn't really saying much. All you are doing is reducing calories from fat and adding back a small amount of protein where the carbs were. So you're eating less calories, but the protein is a little more satiating than the carbs; the exchange of protein for carbs is more filling. The truth is, neither carbs nor fat are your enemy, but the amount you eat of them can be.

In modern day society there are a lot of refined sugar filled food choices. These types of foods are low volume so they don't fill you up, but they are high in calories so these foods periodically add up to a much higher calorie lifestyle.

For most people, eating highly refined carbs leads them to obesity simply because they aren't paying attention to the high amounts of calories they are consuming over the period of a day, a week, and a month. Carbs aren't the enemy; high calorie, low satiating foods combined with inactivity, that's where our problem is.

Don't stop eating carbs to try to lose weight - just pay attention to the carb sources you're using and either eat smaller portions of them or change them to lower calorie versions and more nutrient-dense versions.

Myth #9

"Fat makes you fat."

Again, we need to look at overall calories, calories vs. food volume, and satiation. I know it would be easy to say eating fat makes you fat, sadly that is not valid. Here is the thing my friend: one carb is 4 calories, one gram of protein is 4 calories, and one gram of fat is 9. That doesn't mean that fat is evil, or that fat makes you fat. It just means that per gram, fat thermodynamically is twice as dense as a carb or a gram of protein.

There isn't any really bad way of eating - you always need to look at the context of a nutrition statement before you marry it. It's all about the amount and volume in food size and weight vs. the amount of calories in it.

The reason that fat has a bad name is that some food sources are very low volume but contain high amounts of calories. Things like butter, peanut butter, cheese and oils are very high in calories per gram. For instance, 2 tablespoons (32 grams) of peanut butter is around 190 calories, 16 grams of fat, 8 carbs, and 7 grams of protein.

One tablespoon of full butter is 100 calories and 11 grams of fat. To put this in perspective lets go to the opposite end of the spectrum and show you an example of a very low-calorie food item per gram. So raw spinach leaves are about 7 calories per 32 grams, one carb, one gram of protein and a trace amount of fat.

You would need to eat 815 grams of spinach leaves to get the same amount of calories as 32 grams of peanut butter. That's a lot of leaves. So you see, fat doesn't make you fat, there's simply a lot more calories in oil, butter, and dairy than in other foods. This doesn't mean not to eat them; it just means pay attention to how much peanut butter is on your giant tablespoon.

Myth #10

"Zero calorie foods exist."

If a food or beverage has less than 5 calories per serving, it is legal to put zero calories on the label. Yes, that's right. Every food or drink advertising 0 calories doesn't really have 0 calories.

For example, a food could literally have 3.4 calories per serving, with 100 servings in the box. You would think, hey it's zero calories, but if you eat the whole box of this zero calorie food, you would have eaten 340 calories, surprise mothaf****r.

Zero calorie foods don't exist. This is just manipulated info approved by the FDA because using zero calorie on food labels is a sure way to sell more. Why? Because you will believe it and probably never notice. Zero calorie water flavorings, green teas and seasonings can be great for variety, and they can make your healthy lifestyle more fun and diverse.

However, these products do have calories and can add up if you binge on them. Zero calorie foods are the opposite of high-calorie foods, so you can eat a little more of them regarding volume, but they don't really have zero calories, so tread lightly.

Myth #11

"Fat loss supplements that help you lose 30 pounds in 30 days."

If you ever see that written anywhere, kill it with fire. First of all, unless you're morbidly obese, you won't lose 30 pounds in 30 days unless you stop eating altogether. Even if you could lose that much weight that quickly, you wouldn't want to. That sort of starvation can have negative permanent effects both mentally and physically.

The main reason supplements work is because of one word: "placebo." People eat up the marketing and believe in their minds that with this weight loss product, they will lose weight. So they do.

All weight loss products are nothing more than stimulants and thermogenics that make you sweat a lot, get headaches, increase your heart rate, make you dizzy and more fun stuff. My advice: don't take fat loss supplements, just put in the work at the gym and be consistent with your macronutrient numbers.

Myth #12

"Turning fat into muscle."

This is one of the most frustrating myths in the Health & Fitness industry; I cringe when someone asks me how to turn fat into muscle. Fat has an entirely different biochemical makeup. Muscle tissue and fat are not interchangeable. Fat can only be stored as energy or burned as energy; fat can't turn into muscle, it's impossible.

The closest thing to this is the fact that you can lose fat in a weight loss phase, and then go on a lean muscle gaining phase where you regain muscle in place of the fat. Eventually, over time you can have more muscle and less fat, but you can never directly replace one with the other.

Please don't go gaining a bunch of fat because you want to turn it into muscle. Doing so will only make it 10 times harder on you when it comes time to get lean and lose the fat.

Myth #13

"Sweat is fat crying."

When you're a fitness baby, and someone posts a fit girl picture with this quote written over it on your Facebook news feed, you become super amped up! Yes, time to go make my fat cry.

Marketers are great at making sweating out fat look incredibly sexy to consumers. The truth is fat doesn't cry when you sweat. Sorry, fat is probably laughing at you for thinking it's crying. The only reason that athletes use sweat suits is to make weigh-ins; as soon as they weigh in, they consume water and get all of that weight back in a couple of hours.

Here is something you may want to know: when someone claims they lost 25 pounds in 30 days, over 10 pounds of that is from water manipulation and a couple pounds of that is probably from lower food volume. Less than half of the 25 pounds lost was actual "fat loss."

Sweat is one of the body's natural defense systems that deploys against heat to keep body temperature regulated. When your body is actively working to regulate its temperature in extreme heat or extreme cold, your body does burn a little more calories to regulate its temperature.

The truth is, sweat doesn't have any direct connection to actual fat loss. It's just your body's cooling mechanism. One could argue that there is a correlation, but I would argue that just because something correlates doesn't mean it causes.

Myth #14

"Carb or calorie cycling to jump start the metabolism."

You can't jump start your metabolism - your metabolism isn't this inefficient 90's Honda that you just put nitrous in to make go faster. Carb cycling doesn't change your metabolism. There are a couple reasons that carb cycling became popular. With carb cycling, you can prioritize certain days, for instance, you can place your higher carb days on the more demanding lifting days like a high volume leg day.

Some people like to place their high carb days right before a challenging day so that they wake up on race day/demanding day energized and ready. You can also use carb cycling to be in a caloric deficit on some days and burn fat, and be on a caloric surplus on other days and build some muscle.

Carb cycling is also used with bodybuilders that are extremely lean pre-contest, who need a higher carb day for mental sanity, to help preserve muscle, and to provide a small buffer on the negative effects getting really lean has on their hormones.

The thing is, carb cycling can be very useful and

has many different uses and applications, but it doesn't jumpstart your metabolism.

Myth #15

"Use higher reps to get shredded/lean."

Using higher reps is fine, the problem is that most people have the idea that when they go high in reps that they can use little baby weights that don't challenge them; this is where the problem arises.

High reps are fine, and great, I have nothing against them whatsoever. I even use high reps frequently myself. The issue is that physiologically, the higher that most individuals go in reps, the lower their intensity goes. Most people that do 20+ rep sets aren't at an intensity level of 90% or higher. Most of them are actually at about 50-75% intensity, which means they could do much more than they're doing.

The amount of energy you expend on a given exercise is not based off only reps - energy expenditure on weight training is based off total volume and intensity levels. Weight x Reps x sets + how close you get to max effort on every set. It's not about high or low reps, it's about the big picture.

Just because you're doing high reps doesn't mean you're burning more calories than someone doing less reps; their exercise may be more intense than yours. High reps have their place, but they don't directly burn more fat. You need to look at the context of the high reps to understand if your exercise is efficient. By this, I mean your intensity and volume.

Myth #16

"When you eat before bed, food stores as fat."

This is not true whatsoever. Eating food before bed doesn't make you fat or store your food as fat. Again, it's all about total calories and macronutrients for the day. It's more about how much rather than when.

The reason that this philosophy even became a thing is because there were studies conducted on overweight people. These overweight people typically snacked the most at night; some binged, but they all overate at night. This doesn't mean eating at night is bad, it just means that their overall caloric intake was way too high and the extra snacking or binging at night contributed to the surplus of calories these people were in.

Personally, I like to eat little or no breakfast, a medium sized meal for lunch, a small snack pre-workout, and a giant dinner feast. I have done this for years and lost tons of cumulative weight doing so. This approach helps me never to go to bed hungry. Going to bed hungry is the #1 cause of binge eating or the binge and purge syndrome.

In my opinion, thinking breakfast is crucial and late dinner is bad is setting everyone up for failure mentally. Eating at night is actually very helpful for most people because nobody likes to go to bed hungry, don't be about that life.

Myth #17

"Doing direct abdominal work will burn belly fat and get you better abs."

Spot fat reduction "DOESN'T WORK." It's great to work on your core but don't expect to burn belly fat because of it. Want to burn belly fat? Concentrate on your diet and nutrition, be on a caloric deficit, do your big 3 compound movements i.e. squat, bench press, and deadlift. Stop doing any exercises for the purpose of fat burning. Instead, do them to strengthen the muscles.

Stronger, more stable muscles burn more calories because you're lifting more weight and recruiting more muscle activation than a smaller, less mobile muscle. Building strength, muscle, stability, and mobility - that's what you want to focus on, not silly spot reduction fat loss.

Lose body fat, increase strength and stability on core lifts and stay consistent. Contrary to popular belief, getting abs if you have never had abs takes time, as well as some serious work and dedication. Get the words "six pack shortcuts" out of your vocabulary - there are no shortcuts for hard work.

Myth #18

"The 30-minute anabolic window."

I hate this myth because people get so stressed out about getting their protein shake in. The thing is, there is no need to stress - the anabolic window lasts days, not minutes. If you lost your gains and muscle from not eating protein immediately after your workout, we would all be in some serious trouble.

The "anabolic window," so to speak, can last anywhere from 1 to 3 days and in some cases even 4. Basically, if you work out more than 2-3 days a week, you're living in an anabolic house; forget about the window! You're inside the house of the window.

With this said, there are some exceptions to this when it comes to dieting and being on a caloric deficit. If you have just finished your workout and you feel beat and you need fuel, EAT! But don't worry about losing your gains if something stops you from eating a post workout meal immediately after your workout.

The leaner you get and the longer you're on a caloric deficit, the more beneficial it is to schedule meals pre and post workout purposefully; this is because of the fact that when you are on a caloric deficit for a prolonged period of time and you get really lean, your energy levels will be a little lower.

When losing weight and getting lean, maintaining gym performance is crucial, so you want to schedule your meals in a way that provides you with the most energy for your workouts.

Myth #19

"Eat double your bodyweight in protein to get shredded and build muscle."

First of all, when it comes to macronutrients, i.e. protein, fat and carbs, there is no one size fits all ratio for everyone. The only way to truly figure out what macro ratio works best for you, takes years of trial and error.

I am not saying that you will never understand how many of which macros you need to perform at your best. What I am saying is that it takes some time for each individual to figure that out.

Protein is a very important macronutrient; it's what rebuilds your muscles and the rest of your bodily tissues; even skin, bone, and hair. Protein is the building block of life. Protein also helps you retain muscle when losing body fat and even helps you lose body fat due to the heat dissipation of protein

The thing is, while protein is awesome and we need

it, too much is bad. Too much protein can lead to upset stomach, high acid levels in the body, digestive problems and kidney issues. Now a good range to stick between with your protein is .8-1.2 times your bodyweight in grams of protein per day.

Personally, I am around .9 grams per pound of bodyweight and sometimes even less, and I have had some of the best results ever doing this regarding both fat loss and muscle gain. Now some people do well over 1.2 grams per pound of bodyweight, but that's rare, and like I said, it takes years to truly figure this stuff out for yourself.

A lot of people eat a little more protein when dieting because of the satiating effect it has; it keeps you more full than carbs, but you still need a balanced amount of carbs as well as fats. Every macronutrient plays a role in performance, health and weight loss, so don't become obsessed with one macronutrient or demonize any others.

Myth #20

"Grain products such as bread, pasta, and rice will make you fat."

While these are higher calorie carb sources than veggies, they don't just magically make you fat when you eat them. If some of your daily carbs come from these foods, it won't affect your overall caloric expenditure at the end of the day.

Here is the thing: you want to look more towards the less refined versions of these foods to obtain your nutrients. Whole grain breads, whole grain pastas and brown rice. These versions of the foods have dietary fiber, iron, and many B vitamins. These are things that you need;

the refined versions aren't evil but they aren't actually helping you get any of the necessary nutrients you need.

Weight loss comes down to macros; fat, carb and protein. But you also need your micros like iron and B vitamins. It's not bad to eat refined foods every once in a while; you won't die if you eat refined bread and pasta at a family get together, so don't stress it, enjoy life. Healthy eating and losing weight doesn't have to be hard, stressful or make you anti-social.

Myth #21

"Everyone that gets really shredded is on drugs."

This is not so much of a rumor but more of a philosophy of the ignorant. Some people think that to get really lean, you need drugs. This is simply not the case. It takes heart, dedication, and hard work.

Most people can't fathom the work ethic it takes to develop a beautiful physique. I have gotten to 6% body fat with nothing more than hard work with the weights, cardio, counting macros and my morning coffee. No, I am not genetically gifted with an excellent metabolism. I was a skinny fat kid; at 12, I could not do half a pullup, could not squat or I would fall over, and couldn't do but a couple of bad form pushups.

It took me over 8 years to get my body to the point where I could maintain visible abs year-round. Getting shredded isn't easy, but it is possible and not complicated. Getting super lean is about grinding and digging. It's not about drugs. Not everyone in life takes shortcuts, nothing good comes easy, and what comes easy is also easy to lose. The body will go where the mind takes it.

ACKNOWLEDGMENTS

I would like to acknowledge all of the people who have inspired me on YouTube, who I watch on a weekly and daily basis.

First of all, Christian Guzman, if you don't know who he is, look him up. This guy has been my main source of inspiration for years, in business and building a fitness brand, awesome guy. Secondly, Chris Jones, the man has been at it for a long time and gives a ton of valuable advice daily. I learned a lot from him earlier on in my fitness career. Chris Jones had a lot to do with the inspiration of my subchapter "bulking on a budget."

I would also like to thank Matt Ogus for all of his valuable YouTube content, this man is a beast. He gets absolutely shredded and looks half natty when he competes in bodybuilding shows. And he put Chipotle on the map in terms of the go to post workout restaurant.

Want to lean about macro nutrients in video format? Ogus is another great source. Further, Ogus is the reason I found Jeff Alberts from team 3DMJ. I would like to thank Jeff for all that he taught me over the year of us working together; Jeff is a fantastic contest prep coach! I would like to thank Raymond, the online coach for being a source of daily motivation for me and many others. He is known as the Online Coach, and has a great work ethic and his focus is to motivate, inspire, and teach.

Let me also thank Maxx Chewning for being Maxx Chewning. This guy is one of the most relatable fitness YouTubers out there. Maxx is pure entertainment for me and is a damn beast on the deadlift. I have learned a lot from Maxx just in terms of deadlift technique, great guy!

Last but not least, I would like to thank Nick Wright, who brought me into the YouTube fitness world. Nick had the first Fitness YouTube channel that I started watching back when I was 14. Nick is the godfather of fitness YouTube vloggers! If not for Nick, my life would never have been the same. If I wouldn't have stumbled upon Nick at 14, I may not have found all of these sources of inspiration.

There are many other people that I pay close attention to for learning purposes, like Dr. Layne Norton, Eric Helms, Alan Aragon, Lyle McDonald and many, many more. I owe it to all of them. Seeds of inspiration come in many places; they must be recognized and acknowledged.

Christian
Chris
Matt
Coach
Maxx
Nick

WANT TO LINK UP?

Want to be coached by me? Let's make some GAINZ

Check out our 15-week Alpha 100 Program

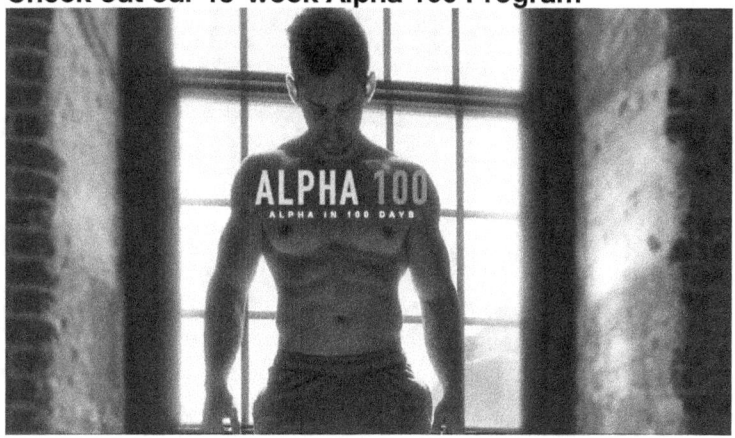

Subscribe to my YouTube channel
Reach out to me on Facebook
DM me on IG
Snap Me @jordanbiaretch
Tweet Me

Email me @Jordanfitness44@gmail.com (serious coaching inquires only)

P.S Thanks gain for taking the time to better yourself. It means the world to me as a writer to be able to affect your life in a positive way.

All Love

www.ingramcontent.com/pod-product-compliance
Lightning Source LLC
Chambersburg PA
CBHW070102290526
45789CB00005B/1895